SURGERY - PROCEDURES, COMPLICATIONS, AND RESULTS

ADVANCES IN SURGICAL PROCEDURES

SURGERY - PROCEDURES, COMPLICATIONS, AND RESULTS

Additional books in this series can be found on Nova's website under the Series tab.

Additional e-books in this series can be found on Nova's website under the e-book tab.

SURGERY - PROCEDURES, COMPLICATIONS, AND RESULTS

ADVANCES IN SURGICAL PROCEDURES

MIRIAM FIGUEROA
EDITOR

NOVA BIOMEDICAL
New York

Library of Congress Cataloging-in-Publication Data

ISBN: 978-1-63482-461-3
Library of Congress Control Number: 2015934863

Published by Nova Science Publishers, Inc. † New York

Contents

Preface

This book presents new research in ambulatory surgery, and discusses advances in other surgical procedures. The topics discussed include ambulatory surgery as well as breast reconstruction, thyroid goitre surgery, and midface lift surgery.

Chapter 1 - Many surgical procedures are performed by ambulatory surgery and account for around 60-70% of all surgical procedures.

The ideal anesthesia in an outpatient setting should offer a smooth, rapid onset of action, produce intraoperative amnesia and analgesia, provide optima surgical conditions with short recovery times, and have no adverse effects.

One of the factors determining the speed of anesthesia recovery is the anesthetic technique used.

Although local and regional anesthesias are anesthetic techniques that are increasingly used for ambulatory surgery because they allow fast recovery, general anesthesia continues to be the most widely employed anesthetic technique.

Inhalation anesthesia is the cornerstone of modern anesthetic practice. New short-acting inhalation anesthetics (e.g., desflurane and sevoflurane) offer fast recovery from anesthesia. However, with the introduction of propofol and new supply systems (e.g., target-controlled infusion), interest in total intravenous anesthesia is growing.

Postoperative pain and vomiting are two factors that usually delay patient recovery and hospital discharge. Identifying those patients at greater risk of postoperative nausea and vomiting may help modify the anesthetic technique used and to use a suitable perioperative prophylaxis.

Older patients and those with a higher classification according to the American Society of Anesthesiologists are at increased risk of perioperative complications. However, deaths related to ambulatory surgery or anesthesia are extremely rare. Some studies have described several complications, but only in 0.08% of cases e.g., myocardial infarction, stroke, pulmonary embolism and respiratory failure.

The most frequent intraoperative complications are cardiovascular events, especially hypotension and hypertension. Other less frequent complications include bradycardia, tachycardia and arrhythmia.

Respiratory events are the second most frequent intraoperative complication, as the most common are laryngospasm and bronchospasm. Other more unusual complications include apnea episodes, aspiration, pneumothorax and pulmonary edema.

The complexity of ambulatory surgical procedures is increasing, as is the morbidity of those patients operated as in an outpatient setting. So while selecting patients for ambulatory surgery, it is very important to minimize perioperative complications as much as possible.

Chapter 2 - Ambulatory surgery is constantly being updated, and is becoming more numerous interventions in this one day regime.

New materials and technological advances will certainly provide a large field of advantages for further proceedings in regimen of short-stay surgery.

New materials:

- Active Sutures: able to release substances at the site where they are applied. For example you sutures with antibiotics.
- Barbed Sutures (self-fixation): no need knotting, facilitating surgery and reducing surgical time.
- Self-gripping Meshes: no need of sutures or glues. This mesh improves thc pain results. It reduces the surgical time.
- Biological synthetics meshes: usefull in hernia repair and in perianal fistulae.
- Laser: useful in hemorrhoids and perianal fistulae.

New techniques:

- Laparoscopy and Open surgery in inguinal hernia repair: TEP, TAPP, using new meshes and barbed sutures, traumatic (absorbable and metallic tackers) and non-traumatic fixation (glues).
- Hernioplasty using new meshes: self-gripping, biological meshes
- Proctology interventions with laser: FILAC, HELP, LHP

All these advances in the surgery field, could improves the results in the ambulatory surgery in our centers. The main reasons are: minor surgical time, the rate of pain is very low, the discharge is in 6-8 hours after the intervention, the quick recovery and functional capacity to work, and the big satisfaction of the patients with these techniques.

Chapter 3 - The concept of day surgery is becoming an increasingly important part of elective surgery worldwide. Relentless pressures to cut costs may constrain clinical judgments regarding the most appropriate location for a patient's surgical care. Ambulatory surgery in Orthopaedics has shown in our institution to be able to provide good-quality service. There still seems to be potential to increase the proportion of these procedures. Therefore, surgeons and anaesthesiologists must strongly adhere to strict patient selection criteria in order to reduce complications in the immediate postoperative term. The authors expose a revision of more than 10.000 patients during the last twenty years following the protocols of our Ambulatory Surgery Unit. Major complications recorded in our revision were minimal without any mortal case. Unplanned overnight admission rate of 0.14% was achieved and a high rate of ambulatory substitution in procedures studied was registered.

Chapter 4 - The abdominal flap is the most common method of autologous breast reconstruction worldwide. Advocates argue the predictability and ability to create a more natural breast mound exceed that of implant based reconstruction. The transverse rectus abdominis (TRAM) flap has evolved from a pedicle flap to a free myocutaneous flap, and now to a deep inferior epigastric perforator (DIEP) flap as microsurgery technique and skill has improved. Multiple recipient vessels have been used historically including the thoracodorsal, lateral thoracic, thoracoacromial, transverse cervical, and internal mammary vessels. The internal mammary artery (IMA) and vein (IMV) are common recipient vessels in today's practice as the dissection can be done quickly and their medial position allows for medial placement of the reconstructed breast mound. During the oncologic portion of the case the axillary lymph nodes are often sampled with either sentinel lymph node biopsy or variations of axillary lymph node dissections. While the axilla is a major nodal basin for breast tissue drainage some studies report as much as 20% drainage to the internal mammary lymph node basin. The dissection of the internal mammary vessels also affords an opportunity to sample internal mammary lymph nodes that may significantly alter cancer staging and treatment. Traditionally, the anastomosis from the free flap to the IMA and IMV is performed in an antegrade manner with a single artery and vein. However, when additional inflow or outflow is needed an additional anastomosis can be performed in the same zone with retrograde anastomosis to the IMA and IMV with success. While the free TRAM is currently the gold standard in autologous breast reconstruction, pre-existing abdominal scars are often a deterrent to the reconstructive surgeon given concern for potential ischemic complications. Techniques involving flap design modification and supercharging or turbocharging the flaps with additional anastomoses from contralateral deep inferior epigastric vessels or superficial inferior epigastric vessels provides the reconstructive surgeon with tools for successfully managing potential problems associated with abdominal scars.

Often clinical analysis of bleeding flap edges is sufficient for assessing flap viability intraoperatively; however, new imaging modalities involving intraoperative laser-assisted indocyanine green (ICG) angiography are also being used as an adjunct to assess tissue perfusion. Other vascular imaging studies such as computed tomography angiography (CTA) are increasingly being used preoperatively to assist with perforator identification and free flap planning. The techniques discussed within this chapter highlight recent advances in perforator based microsurgery, the reconstructive surgeon's potential contribution to breast cancer staging, strategies for managing abdominal scars in abdominal based free tissue breast reconstruction, and the use of vascular imaging for the reconstructive surgeon. These techniques and tips help the reconstructive surgeon to provide excellent and predictable results while limiting complications.

Chapter 5 - Thyroidectomy for goitres can often be challenging, but this is especially apparent for large and difficult goitres. These can often reach very large sizes prior to surgical intervention, and may also extend into, and adhere to, surrounding structures. This makes the surgery more exigent, and increases the risk of damaging major structures inadvertently, including the recurrent laryngeal nerve and parathyroid glands. In this chapter, the authors describe the optimal pre-operative management, including essential imaging to assess the thyroid, and investigations necessary for careful operative planning. The authors describe the operation for such glands in a logical manner, and incorporate techniques and advances which make the surgery more straightforward, and allow the surgeon to carefully identify and preserve vital structures. Further, the authors describe how to approach specific complications resulting from surgery for large goitres, including both intra-operative techniques and post-operative care.

Chapter 6 - *Background:* Since the invention of the first barbed (short) suture by Sulamanidze in the late 1990s, facial soft tissue lifting with subdermal sutures has a significant attraction for physician and patient alike.

This study aimed to describe the authors' experience and the office techniques they have adopted to counteract the descent and laxity of facial soft tissues.

Methods: A retrospective chart review was performed during a period of 15 Months, from March 2013 to June 2014. The procedure was performed in 131 patients under local anesthesia using 2-0 absorbable polylactic sutures with 4 polylactic cones in their distal section (Silhouette Lift, Irvine, California).

The face was marked preoperatively to determine the appropriate vector of the thread and its two end exit points. The results were assessed objectively using serial photography with Canfield Camera System and subjectively according to patient assessment. Complications also were recorded.

Results: All but two patients were satisfied with the outcomes after treatment. Consensus ratings by two independent surgeons found that objective outcomes were divided among "excellent," "good," and "fair." The postoperative course was uneventful except for two patients who presented with major hematoma and another patient who had minor skin dimpling. These three complicated cases were resolved spontaneously without any surgical interventions.

Conclusions: The advantages of this technique are its simplicity, the fact that it produces no traumatic effects, and the fact that it can be performed with local anesthetic, reducing surgical time over current approaches.

In: Advances in Surgical Procedures
Editor: Miriam Figueroa
ISBN: 978-1-63482-461-3

Chapter 1

Ambulatory Surgery: Anesthetic Management and Complications

Monica del-Rio-Vellosillo[1*]
and Jose Javier Garcia-Medina[2†]
[1]Senior Consultant Anesthetist, Department of Anesthesia,
University Hospital Virgen de la Arrixaca, El Palmar, Murcia, Spain
[2]Senior Consultant, Department of Ophthalmology, University Hospital
Reina Sofia, Murcia, Spain and Associate Professor, Department of
Ophthalmology and Optometry, University School of Medicine,
University of Murcia, Murcia, Spain

Abstract

Many surgical procedures are performed by ambulatory surgery and account for around 60-70% of all surgical procedures.

The ideal anesthesia in an outpatient setting should offer a smooth, rapid onset of action, produce intraoperative amnesia and analgesia, provide optima surgical conditions with short recovery times, and have no adverse effects.

One of the factors determining the speed of anesthesia recovery is the anesthetic technique used.

* Email address: monicadelriov@hotmail.com.
† Email address: josegarciam@yahoo.com.

Although local and regional anesthesias are anesthetic techniques that are increasingly used for ambulatory surgery because they allow fast recovery, general anesthesia continues to be the most widely employed anesthetic technique.

Inhalation anesthesia is the cornerstone of modern anesthetic practice. New short-acting inhalation anesthetics (e.g., desflurane and sevoflurane) offer fast recovery from anesthesia. However, with the introduction of propofol and new supply systems (e.g., target-controlled infusion), interest in total intravenous anesthesia is growing.

Postoperative pain and vomiting are two factors that usually delay patient recovery and hospital discharge. Identifying those patients at greater risk of postoperative nausea and vomiting may help modify the anesthetic technique used and to use a suitable perioperative prophylaxis.

Older patients and those with a higher classification according to the American Society of Anesthesiologists are at increased risk of perioperative complications. However, deaths related to ambulatory surgery or anesthesia are extremely rare. Some studies have described several complications, but only in 0.08% of cases e.g., myocardial infarction, stroke, pulmonary embolism and respiratory failure.

The most frequent intraoperative complications are cardiovascular events, especially hypotension and hypertension. Other less frequent complications include bradycardia, tachycardia and arrhythmia.

Respiratory events are the second most frequent intraoperative complication, as the most common are laryngospasm and bronchospasm. Other more unusual complications include apnea episodes, aspiration, pneumothorax and pulmonary edema.

The complexity of ambulatory surgical procedures is increasing, as is the morbidity of those patients operated as in an outpatient setting. So while selecting patients for ambulatory surgery, it is very important to minimize perioperative complications as much as possible.

Introduction

Ambulatory surgery is one of the main areas of anesthesia and surgical practice, and comprises between 60-70% of all procedures [1, 2]. The result of increased limited resources, together with a bigger older population, mean having to place much more emphasis on seeking efficiency and less economic expenditure in medical resources [1].

This type of surgery offers certain benefits for patients, besides monetary saving. It lowers the risk of nosocomial infections and allows patients to recover in a comfortable environment with their family without disrupting their daily routine, which facilitates the cure process and reduces postoperative discomfort [3]. As some authors have demonstrated, this situation is remarkable for the elderly as they suffer cognitive dysfunctions and stress events more often during the first weeks of the postoperative period [4].

Careful patient selection is important to avoid adverse perioperative events. The selection criteria are surgical-, anesthetic- based, and are related to each patient´s characteristics and social environment [5, 6]. Surgical criteria include those patients who do not need any complex preoperative preparations, with no major anatomic or blood volume loss (< 500 mL), require simple postoperative care and no subsequent parenteral treatment, and whose postoperative pain is managed by oral pain medication. Anesthetic criteria include the surgical procedures lasting less than 90 minutes. Patients are catalogued according to the American Society of Anesthesiologists (ASA) I, II and stable III, and can also be considered ASA IV for surgical procedures with local anesthesia. As regards patient characteristics, they need to be cooperative, responsible and have the capacity to understand oral and written orders. Furthermore, the possibility of disposing of responsible adult care when allowed home and during the first 24 h of the postoperative period is also necessary.

One of the important factors that determines patient recovery speed is the anesthetic technique used [2]. Although the use of local and regional anesthesia is increasing in ambulatory surgery as they allow quick patient recovery [7], general anesthesia is still the most widely used anesthetic technique [8, 9]. With the development of new anesthetics drugs, the impulse of multimodal analgesia and antiemetic therapy has extended the ambulatory surgery field [1].

Anesthetic Management

The main goal of ambulatory surgery is to provide smooth surgical anesthesia with rapid onset of action that produces suitable analgesia and intraoperative amnesia. It should also provide quick emergence and recovery, rapid patient rotation at low cost to finally end in a safe hospital discharge with few adverse effects [10].

The quality of anesthetic management includes measures that do not cause further damage to patients, facilitates the best working conditions for surgeons, provides an optimal perioperative care and helps process algorithms to achieve the best clinical results [11].

New anesthetic techniques, short-term anesthetic drugs and analgesics, as well as the development of new anesthetic monitoring equipment, have contributed to make patient recovery quicker [1]. However, all these factors have combined to increase patient costs. Even so, the cost of anesthetic drugs is below 6% of perioperative costs [11]. These costs lower as they also follow economic benefits such as: being able to perform several surgical procedures in the same operative time; a shorter recovery process; fewer staffing requirements.

The choice of the anesthetic technique to be undertaken must be adapted to patient needs, and also to the kind of ambulatory surgery. Premedication, anesthetic, analgesic and antiemetic drugs, and the cardiovascular, hormonal and fluid therapy therapies used will influence the quick recovery of those patients who have undergone ambulatory surgery [12].

Preoperative Medication

Premedication is administered to produce sedation, reduce anxiety, optimize intraoperative hemodynamic stability and cut postoperative side effects without prolonging recovery from anesthesia [13].

Benzodiazepines are the most frequently used drugs for this purpose since small doses improve the perioperative fast-tracking process by reducing anxiety and its complications, as well as improving patient comfort and satisfaction [14]. However, small doses of midazolam which provide anxiolysis and anterograde amnesia, could delay patients from being discharged [15]. Other drugs like β-blockers and α2-agonists, are becoming more popular due to their anesthetic and analgesic-sparing effects [16, 17].

Premedication with α2-agonists, clonidine and dexmedetomidine has been associated with a reduced use of opioid analgesics, postoperative nausea and vomiting (PONV), and intraoperative blood loss [17-19]. The inhibitory effects of these α2-agonists in the sympatho-adrenergic and hypothalamo-pituitary stress response provide glucose control in patients with type 2 diabetes and cut the incidence of ischemic heart disease after surgery [20-22].

β-blockers (e.g., atenolol and esmolol) suppress the increase in circulating catecholamines induced by surgery and prevent cardiovascular events in elderly patients. The anesthetic and analgesic-sparing effects of β-blockers in ambulatory surgery allow quick recovery from anesthesia and cut postoperative side effects (e.g., PONV) [23].

Peripheral Nerve Blockade

A peripheral nerve block (PNB) shares many features of an ideal anesthesia for ambulatory surgery, and provides surgical anesthesia and analgesia at the specific surgical intervention site with few side effects. Administration of long-term local anesthetics is an appealing anesthetic alternative for outpatients [24, 25], and provides a suitable anesthesia and prolonged postoperative analgesia [1].

Placement of perineural catheters with ultrasound guidance as opposed to neurostimulation has proved more effective for treating pain during the first 24 h [26]. Furthermore, ultrasound guidance cuts the number of punctures in patients, makes inserting the catheter much quicker, diminishes vascular punctures, and reduces failing blocks and patient discomfort [27, 28]. It is unclear and has not been scientifically determined whether ultrasound techniques minimize the volume of local anesthetic required besides other non ultrasound block techniques [29].

Determining the concentration of the local anesthetic to be used with this technique is important to strike a balance between pain relief and maintaining appropriate mobility of the operated limb since local anesthetics can affect motor function [30]. Yet for the time being, the optimal regime of the local anesthetic used remains unclear. It would appear that continuous perfusion of local anesthetic combined with on-demand patient-controlled boluses could maximize pain control, and there is some evidence that it improves safety of patients and improves side effects. However, the use of low local anesthetic concentrations does not always correlate with a lower degree of motor block [31-35].

Other drugs have been combined with local anesthetics to increase the speed with which the block begins, to prolong its duration, and to increase intensity and success, while the possibility of toxicity from local also lowers at the same time. Evidence-based studies support the combined use of epinephrine or clonidine together with local anesthetics to delay the systemic absorption of local anesthetics [36-38].

This anesthetic technique acts in a specific place, has few side effects, provides excellent surgical conditions, and a superior analgesia compared with systemic opioids. PNB also lowers the surgical stress response, consumption of opioids, and cuts the duration of stays in postanesthesia care units (PACU), and also the incidence of PONV. It can be used in patients with anticoagulant treatment, increases patient satisfaction and facilitates early patient discharge, besides cutting costs [39-48].

Although this anesthetic technique provides a high degree of satisfaction among the patients undergoing ambulatory surgery [25], the advantages of a single puncture of PNB are limited given the duration of long-term local anesthetics (10-24 h) [24-25]. After the resolution of PNB, postoperative pain management is often difficult and unsuitable in an ambulatory setting. In fact a high proportion of patients (22%) continue to suffer pain and require oral opioids for 7 days of the postoperative period.

This anesthetic technique also offers the possibility of placing perineural catheters for the home pump infusion of local anesthetics by providing patients with continuous analgesia to avoid side effects of oral opioids and to offer greater efficiency than these do [49]. So a continuous peripheral nerve block (CPNB) is a technique that prolongs the effect of local anesthetics at the specific site thanks to the possibility of continuing with the administration of local anesthetics, employing analgesia more profoundly, and avoiding the use of opioids and the early regression of the analgesic block [24]. This technique is well-tolerated by patients as side effects, such as toxicity of local anesthetic, infection or permanent nerve damage [50], are infrequent. On occasion, catheters are difficult to remove due to knotting or looping around nervous structures [51, 52]. It is possible to perform this anesthetic technique in a wide range of surgical procedures for both upper and lower limbs: an interscalene block for shoulder surgery; a supraclavicular and infraclavicular block for surgery of the upper arm to the hand; a lumbar plexus block for hip surgery; a femoral nerve block for surgery of the femur and knee; a sciatic nerve block for the posterior thigh, lower leg and foot [41-44, 53].

However, the clear benefits of this technique to manage pain after ambulatory surgery must be balanced against the cost of the equipment and the resources required to manage these systems safety beyond a medical environment.

Central Neuraxial Block

The introduction of atraumatic pencil-point needles with a small gauge has become an appropriate anesthetic technique with outpatients as it provides a quick, safe and profound surgical block, along with the single injection of small doses of local anesthetics [54].

Choice of local anesthetic type is unclear. Bupivacaine can delay the recovery of the motor function and cause urinary retention by delaying patients from being discharged. Nonetheless, some studies have used low doses of bupivacaine to achieve motor block recovery more quickly, which makes it suitable anesthesia [55]. Nowadays, selective spinal anesthesia is often carried out using minimum doses of intrathecal local anesthetic to anesthetize a specific area. In fact some studies have compared this technique with the use of desflurane, and have reported better postoperative pain control and cost effectiveness with spinal anesthesia [56].

Ropivacaine offers the advantage of producing a reduced motor block by allowing patients to start walking about faster than bupivacaine. However, introperative analgesia and muscle relaxation are suboptimal [57].

Short-acting local anesthetics, such as lidocaine, are associated with a higher incidence of transient neurological symptoms (TNSs), and their use in ambulatory surgery has declined [58].

Other short-acting local anesthetics, such as articaine, chloroprocaine, mepivacaine and prilocaine, have been used in ambulatory surgery successfully [59-63]. These local anesthetics are potentially beneficial because they [64]: 1) produce a motor block of shorter duration and less urinary retention compared with long-acting local anesthetics; 2) offer quick recovery; 3) provide a predictable hospital discharge time; 4) entail a reduced risk of transient neurologic symptoms (TNS) compared with lidocaine. Even so, more urinary retention has been described after administering prilocaine and the block is longer than with articaine, which delays patients from being discharged [65]. However, articaine produces faster recovery than prilocaine, although this does not seem to offer significant advantages compared to 2-chloroprocaine [66, 67]. Several studies have also suggested that the recovery time with 2-chloroprocaine is similar to general anesthesia. However, the use of this drug is not approved in all countries [68-72].

It is possible to add an opioid (e.g., fentanyl or sufentanyl) to the spinal anesthesia solution to reduce the side effects of local anesthetics, shorten patient recovery time and prolong analgesia [73]. This produces increased incidence of postoperative nausea and itching [74]. Another adjuvant used in spinal anesthesia is clonidine, but this combination can produce hypotension and prolong patient recovery [75, 76].

The use of epidural anesthesia with a continuous catheter might help control neuraxial block length in ambulatory surgery [1]. Some studies have suggested that epidural anesthesia is associated with less pain during the postoperative period, fewer interventions by nursing staff in the PACU, lower anesthesia costs and more hemodynamic stability [77]. Nonetheless, it has also been associated with prolonged anesthetic time, delays in discharging patients in short-acting surgeries and potential postoperative urinary retention, particularly in the elderly [3].

Although recovery after a central neuroaxial blockade has improved due to the use of low doses of local anesthetic combined with opioids (fentanyl), patient discharge is often unpredictable and prolonged by approximately 2-4 h after its administration in comparison to general or local anesthesia with sedation [1, 78-79].

A central neuroaxial block offers the benefits of being a simple, safe technique which provides suitable surgical anesthesia. Although it has been associated with prolonged induction times for surgery, they are shorter than with PNB. It has advantages over general anesthesia in terms of cutting the incidence of PONV and sedation [1]. Levels of pain are lower and the need to use opioids in PACU is smaller [80]. It does not cut long-term morbidity, but reduces neurological, cardiac and endocrine complications [81]. Spinal anesthesia as an epidural anesthesia may also lead to perioperative hypotension, postoperative urinary retention, postdural puncture headache, dizziness and delay in onset of walking [3, 82, 47].

General Anesthesia

An ideal general anesthesia technique should provide smooth, quick induction, optimum surgical intervention conditions and a quick recovery with minimum or null side effects [2].

Compared to other anesthetics or inhalations drugs, propofol, sevoflurane, desflurane and short-acting opioids, such as remifentanyl and fentanyl, produce an excellent anesthesia with quick recovery, and also reduce postoperative complications (e.g., respiratory complications, such as airway obstruction and hypoxemia) [83]. Discharge times after using these drugs are comparable with regional anesthesia [77]. Nevertheless, general anesthesia has a higher incidence of PONV and implies more costs [84, 85].

Given its unique recovery profile, propofol is considered the hypnotic of choice to anesthetic induction, although it is more expensive than inhalation anesthetics. Other potential benefits of this drug are antiemetic properties and lower incidence of euphoria and tremors on awakening from anesthesia [86]. However, the non irritant properties of sevoflurane also allow a smooth, quick inhalation anesthesia induction [87-89]. Inhalation anesthesia can be used as an alternative to intravenous induction with propofol and neuromuscular blocking agents if access to an intravenous line is difficult, patients fear needles or it is preferable to keep patients in spontaneous ventilation (e.g., patients with a difficult airway).

Inhalation anesthetics allow faster awakening, probably due to its easy titratibility, and has some neuromuscular blocking effects, which could reduce the requirements of neuromuscular blocking agents [90]. Avoiding neuromuscular blocking agents helps good patient recovery. This is because a residual block may cause uncomfortable symptoms (visual disturbances, inability to sit down without support, facial or generalized weakness) which could delay patient discharge [91], and are usually noticed clinically. Furthermore, the use of sevoflurane can prove more economic than propofol infusion [85, 89, 92]. Even so, with the introduction of new delivery systems (e.g., target-controlled infusion), interest in total IV anesthesia (TIVA) is increasing [93]. When sevoflurane is used, the risk of postoperative emesis and worse patient satisfaction increases. This increase in PONV can delay patient discharge and generate an indirect increase in costs [94, 2].

In clinical terms, there are very few differences between desflurane and sevoflurane. Nonetheless, desflurane allows faster awakening from anesthesia, especially among the elderly and the obese [86]. Desflurane is not often used in ambulatory surgery because it causes cough and irritation in airways [95]. Desflurane is also associated with an increase in PONV compared with propofol. Combinations of antiemetic drugs, such as droperidol, metoclopramide and ondansetron, can lower the incidence of PONV when desflurane is employed [96].

Nitrous oxide is widely utilized in ambulatory surgery. It provides analgesia, reduces inhalation and intravenous anesthetic requirements, which are more expensive, and shortens recovery time. Its higher incidence in PONV has been recently challenged. So there is no convincing reason to avoid its use [86]. New technologies also contribute to fast anesthesia recovery, such as electroencephalographic bispectral index monitoring, which allows the titration of general anesthesia and reduces the amount of hypnotic (propofol or volatile) anesthetic used to maintain anesthesia, thereby facilitating early patient awakening [97-100]. Another monitor to measure anesthesia depth is middle latency auditory evoked potential response amplitudes and latency [101, 102]. It may speed up patient discharge, but has no effect on the amount of anesthetic used or emergence time when inhalation anesthesia is employed.

Remifentanyl has a short-acting duration that is independent of infusion duration. It offers improvement over preoperative analgesia and hemodynamic stability with no harmful effects on the patient awakening time, and this drug even shortens this time because it lowers the concentrations of other drugs used. Neither does it increase PONV as other long-acting opioids do. Providing postoperative rescue analgesia due to the absence of a residual analgesia must also be anticipated [86].

Neuromuscular blocking agents are used to ease endotracheal intubation and the surgical field. In ambulatory surgery, short-acting neuromuscular blocking agents (e.g., succinylcholine) or intermediate-acting neuromuscular blocking agents (e.g., rocuronium) should be considered [103, 104]. The use of sugammadex, a synthetic γ cyclodextrin, allows fast recovery from neuromuscular block after administering rocuronium by avoiding the anticholinergics side effects produced with atropine and neostigmine, or with glycopyrrolate and neostigmine. The latter combination is associated with less nausea and vomiting [105]. It also allows faster tracheal extubation and reduces the postoperative respiratory complications caused by residual muscle paralysis [106].

A laryngeal mask airway (LMA) is a useful, effective alternative to endotracheal intubation for airway management in general anesthesia for ambulatory surgery. Its use reduces the incidence of postoperative sore throat, although no differences have been observed in anesthetic requirements, hospital discharge and the incidence of general side effects [107]. However, LMA is inadvisable in patients at risk of regurgitation (gastroesophageal reflux disease, hiatal hernia, prior gastric surgery, obesity), with pharyngeal or laryngeal pathology, or who present failing lung compliance.

Sedation

The objective of sedation is to achieve hypnosis, anxiolysis and amnesia. Furthermore, we must maintain spontaneous patient breathing and avoid emesis. This requires a striking balance between comfort and patient safety, while preventing cardiovascular and respiratory commitment or delaying patient discharge [108].

Although sedation is often offered as a safer anesthetic technique than general anesthesia, this is not often the case as numerous articles on cardiovascular and respiratory adverse events after the sedation technique have been published [109].

It is accepted that the characteristics of an ideal agent for moderate sedation include rapid onset of action, quick recovery of cognitive and physical faculties following the procedure, and a predictable pharmacokinetic and pharmacodynamic profile.

IV sedatives include short-acting drugs such as propofol, benzodiazepines, ketamine, barbiturates, etomidate and dexmedetomidine. Inhalational agents include sevoflurane and nitrous oxide. Common opioids analgesics comprise fentanyl, remifentanyl and alfentanyl [108, 109].

Many anesthesiologists use a combination of several drugs, and it is difficult to decide between an opioid and a hypnotic as the main drug components of sedation to perform painless sedation.

Sedation is used on many occasions as an adjuvant during the infiltration of local anesthesia or regional anesthesia. However, central nervous system, cardiovascular, and respiratory monitoring is necessary to ensure patient safety.

The success of sedation techniques depends on careful patient and procedure selection, patient preparation, appropriate monitoring, and attention to recovery and discharge.

Complications

Unanticipated hospital admissions after ambulatory surgery reflect intraoperative and postoperative complications, with frequency at around 0.3-1.4% [110]. The reason for higher frequency is for surgical complications (38±79%) [111]. In 10±26% of cases, it is due to anesthetic complications, and more frequently to PONV, somnolence or dizziness, and less commonly to aspiration. In 6-17% of cases, it is due to medial causes, a worsened basal clinic situation, like diabetes, angina and sleep apnea, or to postoperative complications, such as dysrhythmias, myocardial infarction or bronchospasm [111].

Patients who have been subjected to general anesthesia are at a 2-7-fold higher risk of hospital readmission. This is related to length of surgery and perioperative complications [1]. The more frequent causes of hospital readmission are bleeding, fever, infection, wound disruption, and urinary retention [1].

Deaths associated with ambulatory surgery or anesthesia are extremely rare [1]. Studies like that carried out by Warner et al. with 38 598 patients, found two deaths caused by myocardial infarction and two others owing to traffic accidents, at 30 days of ambulatory surgery [112]. Thirty-one cases (0.08%) suffered myocardial infarction, stroke, pulmonary embolism and respiratory failure [112].

With increased complexity in surgical procedures and greater patient comorbidity, the selection of patients for ambulatory surgery is a very important step because patients with cardiovascular and respiratory disease, obesity or smoking history are at increased risk of perioperative complications [113]. Old patients and a higher ASA stage are at risk of intraoperative side effects. Cardiovacular events are the commonest introperative side effect in ambulatory surgery [114], these being hypotension and hypertension with rhythm disturbances, such as bradycardia, tachycardia and arrhythmias, and they happen in approximately 1-2% of outpatients [114].

Respiratory disturbances are the second most frequent intraoperative side effect and occur in less than 1% of cases. Laryngospasm and bronchospasm, with or without desaturation, are the more frequent respiratory events. However, apnea episodes, aspiration, pneumothorax and pulmonary edema have also been described. Development relating to intubation (e.g., tooth damage or esophageal intubation) present a low incidence (0.2±0.5%) [1].

Obese patients can have associated comorbidity with difficult venous access and airway maintenance, thus they present more postoperative complications [115].

Old patients are associated with an overall ‘stiffening’ of the heart and vascular system, as well as autonomic nervous system dysfunction, and are at higher risk of hypothermia. Lung compliance and vital capacity decline are important predictors of postoperative lung complications. The number of neurons and reduced cerebral perfusion with age predispose old patients to greater postoperative cognitive dysfunction. Such patients are more sensitive to the central depressant effects of anesthetic drugs. Deterioration of kidney and liver functions affects the metabolism and excretion of lots of drugs. Old people are also more vulnerable to suffer hypoglycemia episodes during the perioperative period [116].

Other complications might come into play, such as a prolonged hospital stay for several reasons. Postoperative pain, together with nausea and vomiting, are important factors that may prolong hospital stays or produce hospital readmission by 3-4 times [117]. Other side effects include cardiovascular events, dizziness or drowsiness, which also prolong hospital stays [1]. The best predictors of a prolonged hospital stay are intraoperative hemoglobin concentration and blood loss [118].

Postoperative stay duration correlates with the frequency of minor or moderately severe complications. These complications do not tend to require hospital admission, but frequently delay patient discharge. Hospital discharge criteria include stable vital signs, orientation, no pain, no nausea or vomiting, and a responsible attendant being available. In addition patients should be able to start walking about, diuresis should commence, and they should tolerate oral fluids. The use of scoring systems can help standardize care and minimize the risk of unanticipated admission. Several scoring systems are available for postanesthetic discharge, such as the Aldrete Scoring System, or the system designed by Chung and Chung in Toronto, similar to Aldrete´s system, which scores patients from 0 to 2 for the five main criteria prior to discharge [119].

General anesthesia is associated with a major incidence of nausea and vomiting (PONV) (10±50%), and certain more painful surgeries (nose, ear, throat, orthopedic and urological surgeries) will require a longer hospital stay [118, 120]. Several factors have been identified for PONV: female sex, history of PONV or motion sickness, nonsmoking status and use of postoperative opioids [121]. Other predictors include type of anesthesia, surgery lasting more than 60 min, major and laparoscopic gynecological surgery, laparoscopic cholecystectomy, intra-abdominal surgery, and middle-ear surgery [123-125]. Hypotension due to inadequate hydration, early walking and movement, and force fluid intake can increase the risk of PONV [126]. Strategies to cut the incidence of PONV include: 1) use of TIVA with propofol which reduces PONV by around 19% [12, 86, 127-131]; 2) use of nitrous oxide is a questioned risk factor of PONV, although it is not as significant as volatile anesthetic agents. Both propofol and inhalation anesthetic agent produce more emesis when they are used with nitrous oxide. No differences among isoflurane, desflurane and sevoflurane have been found for emesis. A drop in PONV by up to 12% has been described when nitrous oxide; 3) minimizing opioids lowers the risk of PONV. Infiltration of local anesthetics, and use of alternative non narcotic analgesics and multimodal anesthetic techniques will reduce the employment of opioid; 4) regional anesthesia is associated with a marked cut in the risk of PONV compared to inhalation-based general anesthesia, thus avoiding exposure to volatile anesthetics and narcotics; 5) minimizing the use of reversal drugs; 6) maintaining adequate patient hydration; 7) multimodal individualized antiemetic treatment

Therefore, identifying these patients will help achieve successful PONV control through a change in the anesthetic technique used, a lower basal risk and a suitable prophylaxis technique.

A wide variety of antiemetic drugs are available for treating PONV, including serotonin antagonists, steroids, dopamine antagonists. Other drugs include antihistamines, anticholinergics, sympathomimetics drugs and neurokinin-1 antagonists [132]. Use of sympatholytic drugs (e.g., esmolol, labetalol), agonist/antagonists, and even ketamine, to control transient autonomic responses during surgery, can reduce PONV because of their anesthetic and opioid-sparing effects [17, 133, 134].

Serotonin antagonists are drugs such as ondansetron, dolasetron, granisetron, and palonosetron. Ondansetron was the first to appear and is the most broadly studied one, whose most frequent side effects include headache, constipation and diarrhea. Doses of 4 mg administered 20-30 min before surgery and finishing the supply of a PONV prophylaxis between 4-6 h post-surgery are recommended [135].

Other drugs used to prevent PONV are steroids, such as dexamethasone. This drug has a slower onset of action, so its administration is recommended immediately after inducing anesthesia. Its exact mechanism is not completely known, although it is thought that steroids inhibit prostaglandin synthesis at the central level and allow endorphin release. It is recommended in doses of 4-8 mg [136, 137].

Among dopamine antagonists, droperidol and haloperidol produce an alpha blockade, so they could produce sedation and extrapyramidal symptoms. However, these side effects do not usually appear with small the doses administered to prevent PONV (0.625/1.25 mg) [135].

Of all these drugs that prevent PONV, the three most commonly used ones are ondansetron 4 mg, dexamethasone 4 mg, and droperidol 1.25 mg, which all have a similar effectiveness on preventing PONV, and the risk is cut up to 26% when any of them is used [127]. The use, or not, of these drugs, and their combination, depend on the risk factors presented by each patient. Hence treatment must be individualized since performing antiemetic prophylaxis in all patients may not be indicated due to the expense and side effects involved [127, 138, 139].

Managing pain with a multimodal approach will allow the better control of postoperative pain and will involve fewer side effects, such as those observed with certain drugs like opioids [140]. We must ensure that patients are discharged from hospital with good pain control.

The drugs used in multimodal analgesia tend to be non steroidal anti-inflammatory drugs (NSAIDs), beta-blockers, N-methyl D-aspartate (NMDA) inhibitors, steroids and alpha-2 agonists, or local anesthetics. Other techniques have also been used: non pharmacological techniques like transcutaneous electrical stimulation and transcutaneous acupoint electrical stimulation [1, 128, 141].

Regarding the use of morphine or fentanyl in ambulatory surgery, fentanyl offers a faster onset of action, but according to some published studies, it does not seem to be associated with faster patient discharge. Most patients required additional analgesia to control pain. However, morphine has been reported to produce better quality analgesia, but has been associated with a higher incidence of nausea and vomiting, especially after discharge [142].

Other factors that can delay patients from being discharged include: sore throat, headache, dizziness and drowsiness [143]. The incidence of sore throat is 12.1%, and this becomes higher with the use of an endotracheal tube compared to LMA (45.4% *vs.* 17.5%, respectively) [144]. Perioperative hydration with 20 mL/kg^{1} of IV isotonic fluid produces fewer postoperative symptoms, like thirst, nausea, dizziness and drowsiness, for the first 24 h of the postoperative time [126].

References

[1] Troy AM, Cunningham AJ. Ambulatory surgery: an overview. *Curr Opin Anaesthesiol.* 2002;15:647-57.

[2] Joshi GP. Inhalational techniques in ambulatory anesthesia. *Anesthesiol Clin North America.* 2003;21:263-72.

[3] White PF, White LM, Monk T, Jakobsson J, Raeder J, Mulroy MF, Bertini L, Torri G, Solca M, Pittoni G, Bettelli G. Perioperative care for the older outpatient undergoing ambulatory surgery. *Anesth Analg.* 2012;114:1190-215.

[4] Canet J, Raeder J, Rasmussen LS, Enlund M, Kuipers HM, Hanning CD, Jolles J, Korttila K, Siersma VD, Dodds C, Abildstrom H, Sneyd JR, Vila P, Johnson T, Munoz CL, Silverstein JH, Nielsen IK, Moller JT. Cognitive dysfunction after minor surgery in the elderly. *Acta Anaesthesiol Scand.* 2003;47:1204-10.

[5] Ministerio de Sanidad y Consumo. Dirección General de Aseguramiento y Planificación Sanitaria. Cirugía Mayor Ambulatoria. Guía de Organización y Funcionamiento. Madrid; Ministerio de Sanidad y Consumo, 1993.

[6] Royal Australasian College of Surgeons, Australian and New Zealand College of Anaesthetists, The Australian Society of Anaesthetists. Day Surgery in Australia. Report and Recommendations of the Australian Day Surgery Council. 2004.

[7] Joshi GP. Recent developments in regional anesthesia for ambulatory surgery. *Curr Opin Anaesthesiol.* 1999;12:643-7.

[8] Joshi GP. Fast tracking in outpatient surgery. *Curr Opin Anaesthesiol.* 2001;14:635-9.

[9] Joshi GP, Twersky RS. Fast tracking in ambulatory surgery. *Ambulatory Surgery*. 2000;8:185-90.

[10] Chikungwa M, Smith I. Controversial issues in ambulatory anesthesia. *Anesthesiol Clin North America*. 2003;21:313-27.

[11] White PF, Watcha MF. Pharmacoeconomics in anaesthesia: what are the issues? *Eur J Anaesthesiol Suppl.* 2001;23:10-5.

[12] White PF, Eng M. Fast-track anesthetic techniques for ambulatory surgery. *Curr Opin Anaesthesiol*. 2007;20:545-57.

[13] White PF. Pharmacologic and clinical aspects of preoperative medication. *Anesth Analg*. 1986;65:963-74.

[14] van Vlymen JM, Sa Rego MM, White PF. Benzodiazepine premedication: can it improve outcome in patients undergoing breast biopsy procedures? *Anesthesiology*. 1999;90:740-7.

[15] Taylor E, Ghouri AF, White PF. Midazolam in combination with propofol for sedation during local anesthesia. *J Clin Anesth*. 1992;4:213-6.

[16] Chia YY, Chan MH, Ko NH, Liu K. Role of beta-blockade in anaesthesia and postoperative pain management after hysterectomy. *Br J Anaesth*. 2004;93:799-805.

[17] Segal IS, Jarvis DJ, Duncan SR, White PF, Maze M. Clinical efficacy of oral-transdermal clonidine combinations during the perioperative period. *Anesthesiology*. 1991;74:220-5.

[18] Aho MS, Erkola OA, Scheinin H. Effect of intravenously administered dexmedetomidine on pain after laparoscopic tubal ligation. *Anesth Analg*. 1991;73:112-8.

[19] Okuyama K, Inomata S, Toyooka H. The effects of prostaglandin E1 or oral clonidine premedication on blood loss during paranasal sinus surgery. *Can J Anesth.* 2005;52:546-7.

[20] Mertes N, Goetters C, Kuhlmann M, Zander JF. Postoperative alpha-2 adrenergic stimulation attenuates protein catabolism. *Anesth Analg*. 1996;82:258-63.

[21] Belhoula M, Ciebiera JP, De La Chapelle A, Boisseau N, Coeurveille D, Raucoules-Aimé M.. Clonidine premedication improves metabolic control in type 2 diabetic patients during ophthalmic surgery. *Br J Anaesth*. 2003;90:434-9.

[22] Wallace AW, Galindez D, Salahieh A, Layug EL, Lazo EA, Haratonik KA, Boisvert DM, Kardatzke D.. Effect of clonidine on cardiovascular morbidity after noncardiac surgery. *Anesthesiology*. 2004;101:284-93.

[23] Zaugg M, Tagliente T, Lucchinetti E, Jacobs E, Krol M, Bodian C, Reich DL, Silverstein JH. Beneficial effects from betaadrenergic blockade in elderly patients undergoing noncardiac surgery. *Anesthesiology*. 1999;91:1674-86.

[24] Klein S. M, Pietrobon R, Nielsen K. C, Warner D. S, Greengrass R. A. Peripheral nerve blockade with longacting local anesthetics, of the Society for Ambulatory Anesthesia. *Anesth Analg*. 2002;94:71-6.

[25] Klein SM, Nielson KC, Greengrass RA, Warner DS, Martin A, Steele SM. Ambulatory discharge after longacting peripheral nerve blockade: 2382 blocks with ropivacaine. *Anesth Analg*. 2002;94:65-70.

[26] Fredrickson M, Ball C, Dalgleish A. A prospective randomized comparison of ultrasound guidance versus neurostimulation for interscalene catheter placement. *Regional Anesth Pain Med*. 2009;34:590-4.

[27] Abrahams M, Aziz M, Fu R, Horn J. Ultrasound guidance compared with electrical stimulation for peripheral nerve block: a systemic review and metaanalysis of randomized controlled trials. *BJA*. 2009;102:408-17.

[28] Mariano E, Loland V, Bellars R, Sandhu NS, Bishop ML, Abrams RA, Meunier MJ, Maldonado RC, Ferguson EJ, Ilfeld BM. Ultrasound guidance versus electrical stimulation for infraclavicular brachial plexus perineural catheter insertion. *J Ultrasound Med*. 2009;28:1211-8.

[29] Duggan E, Beheiry H, Perlas A, Lupu M, Nuica A, Chan VW, Brull R. Minimum effective volume of local anesthetic for ultrasound-guided supraclavicular brachial plexus block. *Regional Anesth Pain Med*. 2009;34:215-8.

[30] Axley M, Horn JL. Indications and management of continuous infusion of local anesthetics at home. *Curr Opin Anaesthesiol*. 2010;23:650-5.

[31] Fisher H, Simanski C, Sharp C, Bonnet F, Camu F, Neugebauer EA, Rawal N, Joshi GP, Schug SA, Kehlet H. A procedure-specific systematic review and consensus recommendations for postoperative analgesia following total knee arthroplasty. *Anaesthesia*. 2008;63:1105-23.

[32] Ilfeld B, Loland V, Gerancher J, Wadhwa AN, Renehan EM, Sessler DI, Shuster JJ, Theriaque DW, Maldonado RC, Mariano ER. The effects of varying local anesthetic concentration and volume on continuous popliteal sciatic nerve blocks: a dual center, randomized, controlled study. *Anesth Analg*. 2008;107:701-7.

[33] Brodner G, Buerkle H, Van Aken H, Lambert R, Schweppe-Hartenauer ML, Wempe C, Gogarten W. Postoperative analgesia after knee surgery: a comparison of three different concentrations of ropivacaine for continuous femoral nerve blockade. *Anesth Analg.* 2007;105:256-62.

[34] Paauwe J, Thomassen B, Weterings J, van Rossum E, Ausems ME. Femoral nerve block using ropivacaine 0.025%, 0.05% and 0.1% effects on the rehabilitation programme following total knee arthroplasty: a pilot study. *Anaesthesia.* 2008;63:948-53.

[35] Ilfeld B, Le LT, Ramjohn J, Loland V, Wadhwa AN, Gerancher JC, Renehan EM, Sessler DI, Shuster JJ, Theriaque DW, Maldonado RC, Mariano ER. The effects of local anesthetic concentration and dose on continuous infraclavicular nerve blocks: a multicenter, randomized, observer-masked, controlled study. *Anesth Analg.* 2009; 108:345-50.

[36] Thornton PC, Grant SA, Breslin DS. Adjuncts to local anesthetics in peripheral nerve blockade. *Int Anesthesiol Clin.* 2010;48:59-70.

[37] Bernards CM, Kopacz DJ. Effect of epinephrine on lidocaine clearance in vivo: a microdialysis study in humans. *Anesthesiology.* 1999;91:962-8.

[38] Eisenach JC, DeKock M, Klimscha W. Alpha(2)-adrengic agonists for regional anesthesia. A clinical review of clonidine (1984 to 1995). *Anesthesiology.* 1996;85:655-74.

[39] Rawal N, Axelsson K, Hylander J, Allvin R, Amilon A, Lidegran G, Hallén J. Postoperative patient-controlled local anesthetic administration at home. *Anesth Analg.* 1998;86:86-9.

[40] Ilfeld B, Morey T, Enneking K. Continuous infraclavicular brachial plexus block for postoperative pain control at home. a randomized, double-blinded, placebo-controlled study. *Anesthesiology.* 2002;96:1297-304.

[41] Ilfeld B, Vandenborne K, Duncan P, Sessler DI, Enneking FK, Shuster JJ, Theriaque DW, Chmielewski TL, Spadoni EH, Wright TW. Ambulatory continuous interscalene nerve blocks decrease the time to discharge readiness after total shoulder arthroplasty: a randomized, triple-masked, placebo-controlled study. *Anesthesiology.* 2006;105:999-1007.

[42] Ilfeld B, Morey T, Enneking F. Infraclavicular perineural local anesthetic infusion. *Anesthesiology.* 2004;100:395-402.

[43] 43. Ilfeld B, Morey T, Wang D. Continuous popliteal sciatic nerve block for postoperative pain control at home. *Anesthesiology.* 2002;97:959-65.

[44] Ilfeld B, Ball S, Gearen P. Ambulatory continuous posterior lumbar plexus nerve blocks after hip arthroplasty. *Anesthesiology*. 2008;109:491-501.

[45] Ilfeld B, Le L, Meyer S. Ambulatory continuous femoral nerve blocks decrease time to discharge readiness after tricompartmental total knee arthroplasty. *Anesthesiology*. 2008;108:703-13.

[46] Ilfeld B, Mariano E, Williams B, Woodard JN, Macario A. Hospitalization costs of total knee arthroplasty with a continuous femoral nerve block provided only in the hospital versus on an ambulatory basis: a retrospective, case-control, cost-minimization analysis. *Reg Anesth Pain Med*. 2007;32:46-54.

[47] Capdevila X, Dadure C. Perioperative management for one day hospital admission: regional anesthesia is better than general anesthesia. *Acta Anaesthesiol Belg*. 2004;55 Suppl:33-6.

[48] Hadzic A, Williams BA, Karaca PE, Hobeika P, Unis G, Dermksian J, Yufa M, Thys DM, Santos AC. For outpatient rotator cuff surgery nerve block anesthesia provides superior same-day recovery over general anesthesia. *Anesthesiology*. 2005;102:1001-7.

[49] Apfelbaum J, Chen C, Mehta S, Gan TJ. Postoperative pain experience: results from a national survey suggest postoperative pain continues to be undermanaged. *Anesth Analg*. 2003;97:534-40.

[50] Swenson J, Bay N, Loose E, Bankhead B, Davis J, Beals TC, Bryan NA, Burks RT, Greis PE. Outpatient management of continuous peripheral nerve catheters placed using ultrasound guidance: an experience in 620 patients. *Anesth Analg*. 2006;103:1436-43.

[51] Offerdahl MR, Lennon RL, Horlocker TT. Successful removal of a knotted fascia iliaca catheter: principles of patient positioning for peripheral nerve catheter extraction. *Anesth Analg*. 2004;99:1550-2.

[52] MacLeod D. Knotted peripheral nerve catheter. *Reg Anesth Pain Med*. 2003;28:487-8.

[53] Ilfeld B, Wright T, Enneking K, Vandenborne K. Total elbow arthroplasty as an outpatient procedure using a continuous infraclavicular nerve block at home: a prospective case report. *Regional Anesth Pain Med*. 2006;31:172-6.

[54] Casati A, Cappelleri G, Fanelli G, Borghi B, Anelati D, Berti M, Torri G. Regional anaesthesia for outpatient knee arthroscopy: a randomized clinical comparison of two different anaesthetic techniques. *Acta Anaesthesiol Scand*. 2000;44:543-7.

[55] Valanne JV, Korhonen AM, Jokela RM, Ravaska P, Korttila KK. Selective spinal anesthesia: a comparison of hyperbaric bupivicaine 4 mg versus 6 mg for outpatient knee arthroscopy. *Anesth Analg.* 2001;93:1377-9.
[56] Lennox PH, Chilvers C, Vaghadia H. Selective spinal anesthesia versus desflurane anesthesia in short duration outpatient gynecological laparoscopy: a pharmacoeconomic comparison. *Anesth Analg.* 2002;94:565-8.
[57] Gautier P, De Kock M, Van Steenberge A, Poth N, Lahaye-Goffart B, Fanard L, Hody JL. Intrathecal ropivicaine for ambulatory surgery: a comparison between intrathecal bupivicaine and intrathecal ropivicaine for knee arthroscopy. *Anesthesiology*. 1999;91:1239-45.
[58] Keld DB, Hein L, Dalgaard M, Krogh L, Rodt SA. The incidence of transient neurologicsymptoms (TNS) after spinal anesthesia in patients undergoing surgery in the supine position: hyperbaric lidocaine 5% versus hyperbaric bupivacaine 0.5%. *Acta Anesthesiol Scand.* 2000;44:285-90.
[59] Watson B, Howell V. Spinal anaesthesia: the saviour of day surgery? *Curr Anaesth Crit Care*. 2007;80:96-112.
[60] Förster JG, Rosenberg PH. Revival of old local anesthetics for spinal anesthesia in ambulatory surgery. *Curr Opin Anaesthesiol.* 2011;24:633-7.
[61] Wulf H, Hampl K, Steinfeldt T. Speed spinal anesthesia revisited: new drugs and their clinical effects. *Curr Opin Anaesthesiol.* 2013;26:613-20.
[62] del-Rio-Vellosillo M, Garcia-Medina JJ, Abengochea-Cotaina A, Pinazo-Duran MD. Intrathecal local anaesthetics in ambulatory surgery. *Acta Anaesthesiol Scand*. 2014;58:906.
[63] Camponovo C, Wulf H, Ghisi D, Fanelli A, Riva T, Cristina D, Vassiliou T, Leschka K, Fanelli G. Intrathecal 1% 2-chloroprocaine vs. 0.5% bupivacaine in ambulatory surgery: a prospective, observer-blinded, randomised, controlled trial. *Acta Anaesthesiol Scand.* 2014;58:560-6.
[64] Förster JG. Short-acting spinal anesthesia in the ambulatory setting. *Curr Opin Anaesthesiol*. 2014;27:597-604.
[65] Kreutziger J, Frankenberger B, Luger TJ, Richard S, Zbinden S. Urinary retention after spinal anaesthesia with hyperbaric prilocaine 2% in an ambulatory setting. *Br J Anaesth.* 2010;104:582-6.

[66] Hendriks MP, de Weert CJ, Snoeck MM, Hu HP, Pluim MA, Gielen MJ. Plain articaine or prilocaine for spinal anaesthesia in day-case knee arthroscopy: a double-blind randomized trial. *Br J Anaesth.* 2009;102:259-63.

[67] Förster JG, Kallio H, Rosenberg PH, Harilainen A, Sandelin J, Pitkänen MT. Chloroprocaine vs. articaine as spinal anaesthetics for day-case knee arthroscopy. *Acta Anaesthesiol Scand.* 2011;55:273-81.

[68] Casati A, Fanelli G, Danelli G, Berti M, Ghisi D, Brivio M, Putzu M, Barbagallo A. Spinal anesthesia with lidocaine or preservative-free 2-chlorprocaine for outpatient knee arthroscopy: a prospective, randomized, double-blind comparison. *Anesth Analg.* 2007;104:959-64.

[69] Sell A, Tein T, Pitkänen M. Spinal 2-chloroprocaine: effective dose for ambulatory surgery. *Acta Anaesthesiol Scand.* 2008;52:695-9.

[70] Yoos JR, Kopacz DJ. Spinal 2-chloroprocaine for surgery: an initial 10-month experience. *Anesth Analg.* 2005;100:553-8.

[71] Kouri ME, Kopacz DJ. Spinal 2-chloroprocaine: a comparison with lidocaine in volunteers. *Anesth Analg.* 2004;98:75-80.

[72] Hejtmanek MR, Pollock JE. Chloroprocaine for spinal anesthesia: a retrospective analysis. *Acta Anaesthesiol Scand.* 2011;55:267-72.

[73] Akcaboy ZN, Akcaboy EY, Mutlu NM, Serger N, Aksu C, Gogus N. Spinal anesthesia with low-dose bupivacaine–fentanyl combination: a good alternative for day case transurethral resection of prostrate surgery in geriatric patients. *Rev Bras Anesthesiol.* 2012;6:753-61.

[74] Ben-David B, DeMeo PJ, Lucyk C, Solosko D. A comparison of minidose lidocaine-fentanyl spinal anesthesia and local anesthesia/propofol infusion for outpatient knee arthroscopy. *Anesth Analg.* 2001;93:319-25.

[75] Singh H, Liu J, Gaines GY, White PF. Effect of oral clonidine and intrathecal fentanyl on tetracaine spinal block. *Anesth Analg.* 1994;79:1113-6.

[76] van Tuijl I, Giezeman MJ, Braithwaite SA, Hennis PJ, Kalkman CJ, van Klei WA. Intrathecal low-dose hyperbaric bupivacaine-clonidine combination in outpatient knee arthroscopy: a randomized controlled trial. *Acta Anaesthesiol Scand.* 2008;52:343-9.

[77] Mulroy MF, Larkin KL, Hodgson PS, Helman JD, Pollock JE, Liu SS. A comparison of spinal, epidural, and general anesthesia for outpatient knee arthroscopy. *Anesth Analg.* 2000;91:860-4.

[78] Nair GS, Abrishami A, Lermitte J, Chung F. Systematic review of spinal anaesthesia using bupivacaine for ambulatory knee arthroscopy. *Br J Anaesth*. 2009;102:307-15.

[79] O'Donnell D, Manickam B, Perlas A, Karkhanis R, Chan VW, Syed K, Brull R. Spinal mepivacaine with fentanyl for outpatient knee arthroscopy surgery: a randomized controlled trial. *Can J Anaesth*. 2010;57:32-8.

[80] Liu SS, Strodtbeck WM, Richman JM, Wu CL. A comparison of regional versus general anesthesia for ambulatory anesthesia: a meta-analysis of randomized controlled trials. *Anesth Analg*. 2005;101:1634-42.

[81] Nordquist D, Halaszynski TM. Perioperative multimodal anesthesia using regional techniques in the aging surgical patient. *Pain Res Treat*. 2014;2014:902174.

[82] Auroy Y, Benhamou D, Bargues L, Eccoey C, Falissard B, Mercier FJ, Bouaziz H, Samii K. Major complications of regional anesthesia in France: the SOS Regional Anesthesia Hotline Service. *Anesthesiology*. 2002;97:1274-80.

[83] Georgiou LG, Vourlioti AN, Kremastinou FI, Stefanou PS, Tsiotou AG, Kokkinou MD. Influence of anesthetic technique on early postoperative hypoxemia. *Acta Anaesthesiol Scand*. 1996;40:75-80.

[84] Tang J, Chen L, White PF, Watcha MF, Wender RH, Naruse R, Kariger R, Sloninsky A. Recover profile, costs, and patient satisfaction with propofol and sevoflurane for fast-track office-based anesthesia. *Anesthesiology*. 1999; 91:253-61.

[85] Smith I, Terhoeve PA, Hennart D, Feiss P, Harmer M, Pourriat JL, Johnson IA. A multicentre comparison of the costs of anaesthesia with sevoflurane or propofol. *Br J Anaesth*. 1999;83:564-70.

[86] Dewandre PY. Peroperative management for ambulatory anaesthesia: does the choice of drug matter? *Acta Anaesthesiol Belg*. 2004;55 Suppl:39-40.

[87] Joo HS, Perks WJ. Sevoflurane versus propofol for anesthetic induction: a meta-analysis. *Anesth Analg*. 2000;91:213-9.

[88] Philip BK, Lombard LL, Roaf ER, Drager LR, Calalang I, Philip JH.. Comparison of vital capacity induction with sevoflurane to intravenous induction with propofol for adult ambulatory anesthesia. *Analg Anesth*. 1999; 89:623-7.

[89] Watson KR, Shah MV. Clinical comparison of 'single agent' anaesthesia with sevoflurane versus target controlled infusion of propofol. *Br J Anaesth*. 2000;85:541-6.

[90] Eriksson LI. The effects of residual neuromuscular blockade and volatile anesthetics on control of ventilation. *Anesth Analg*. 1999;89:243-51.

[91] Kopman AF, Yee PS, Neuman GG. Relationship of the train-of-four fade ratio to clinical signs and symptoms of residual paralysis in awake volunteers. *Anesthesiology*. 1997;86:765-71.

[92] Thwaites A, Edmends S, Smith I. Inhalation induction with sevoflurane: a double-blind comparison with propofol. *Br J Anaesth*. 1997;78:356-61.

[93] Tonner PH, Scholz J. Total intravenous or balanced anaesthesia in ambulatory surgery? *Curr Opin Anaesthesiol*. 2000;13:631-6.

[94] Smith I, Thwaites AJ. Target-controlled propofol vs. sevoflurane: a double-blind, randomised comparison in day-case anaesthesia. *Anaesthesia*. 1999;8:745-52.

[95] Mahmoud NA, Rose DJA, Laurence AS. Desflurane or sevoflurane for gynaecological day-case anaesthesia with spontaneous respiration? *Anaesthesia*. 2001; 56:171-4.

[96] Tang J, White PF, Wender RH, Naruse R, Kariger R, Sloninsky A, Karlan MS, Uyeda RY, Karlan SR, Reichman C, Whetstone B. Fast-track office-based anesthesia: a comparison of propofol versus desflurane with antiemetic prophylaxis in spontaneously breathing patients. *Anesth Analg*. 2001;92:95-9.

[97] Nelskyla KA, Yli-Hankala AM, Puro PH, Korttila KT. Sevoflurane titration using bispectral index decreases postoperative vomiting in phase II recovery after ambulatory surgery. *Anesth Analg*. 2001;93:1165-9.

[98] Pavlin DJ, Hong JY, Freund PR, Koerschgen ME, Bower JO, Bowdle TA. The effect of bispectral index monitoring on end-tidal gas concentration and recovery duration after outpatient anesthesia. *Anesth Analg*. 2001;93:613-9.

[99] Gan TJ, Glass PS, Windsor A, Payne F, Rosow C, Sebel P, Manberg P. Bispectral index monitoring allows faster emergence and improved recovery from propofol, alfentanil, and nitrous oxide anesthesia. BIS Utility Study Group. *Anesthesiology*. 1997;87:808-15

[100] Song D, Joshi GP, White PF. Titration of volatile anesthetics using bispectral index facilitates recovery after ambulatory anesthesia. *Anesthesiology*. 1997;87:842-8.

[101] Assareh H, Anderson RE, Uusijarvi J, Jakobsson J. Sevoflurane requirements during ambulatory surgery: a clinical study with and without AEP-index guidance. *Acta Anaesthesiol Scand*. 2002;46:495-9.

[102] Assare H, Anderson RE, Jakobsson J. Sevoflurane requirements during ambulatory surgery: a clinical study of bispectral index and auditory evoked potential guided anaesthesia. *Amb Surg*. 2002;9:207-11.

[103] Schlaich N, Mertzlufft F, Soltesz S, Fuchs-Buder T. Remifentanil and propofol without muscle relaxants or with different doses of rocuronium for tracheal intubation in outpatient anaesthesia. *Acta Anaesthesiol Scand*. 2000;44:720-6.

[104] Murphy GS, Szokol JW, Marymont JH, Avram MJ, Vender JS, Rosengart TK. Impact of shorter-acting neuromuscular blocking agents on fast-track recovery of the cardiac surgery patient. *Anesthesiology*. 2002;96:600-6.

[105] Chhibber AK, Lustik SJ, Thakur R, Francisco DR, Fickling KB. Effects of anticholinergics on postoperative vomiting, recovery and hospital stay in children undergoing tonsillectomy with or without adenoidectomy. *Anesthesiology*. 1999;90:697-700.

[106] Sacan O, White PF, Tufanogullari B, Klein K. Sugammadex reversal of rocuronium-induced neuromuscular blockade: a comparison with neostigmine-glycopyrrolate and edroponium–atrophine. *Anesth Analg*. 2007;104:569-74.

[107] Joshi GP, Inagaki Y, White PF, Taylor-Kennedy L, Wat LI, Gevirtz C, McCraney JM, McCulloch DA. Use of the laryngeal mask as an alternative to the tracheal tube during ambulatory anesthesia. *Anesth Analg*. 1997;85:573-7.

[108] Greenberg CP, De Soto H. Sedation techniques. In: Twersky RS, ed: *The Ambulatory Anesthesia Handbook*. St Louis, MO: Mosby; 1995:301-59.

[109] Philip BK, Minzter BH. Intravenous sedation and monitored anesthesia care. In: White PF, ed. *Ambulatory Anesthesia and Surgery*. Philadelphia, PA: W.B. Saunders; 1997:349-67.

[110] Fortier J, Chung F, Su J. Unanticipated admission after ambulatory surgery: a prospective study. *Can J Anaesth*. 1998;45:612-9.

[111] Twersky R, Fishman D, Homel P. What happens after discharge? Return hospital visits after ambulatory surgery. *Anesth Analg.* 1997;84:319-24.

[112] Warner MA, Shields SE, Shute CG. Major morbidity and mortality within one month of ambulatory surgery and anesthesia. *JAMA.* 1993;270:1437-41.

[113] Chung F, Mezei G, Tong D. Pre-existing medical conditions as predictors of adverse events in day-case surgery. *Br J Anaesth.* 1999;83:262-70.

[114] Duncan PD, Reccan PG, Cohen MM, Tweed WA. The Canadian Four Centre Study of anaesthetic outcomes: are anesthetic complications predictable in day surgical practice? *Can J Anesth.* 1992;39:440-8.

[115] Atkins M, White J, Ahmed K. Day surgery and body mass index: results of a national survey. *Anaesthesia.* 2002;57:180-2.

[116] Aurini L, White PF. Anesthesia for the elderly outpatient. *Curr Opin Anaesthesiol.* 2014;27:563-75.

[117] Chung F, Ritchie E, Su J. Post-operative pain in ambulatory surgery. *Anesth Analg.* 1997;85:808-16.

[118] Junger A, Klasen J, Benson M, Sciuk G, Hartmann B, Sticher J, Hempelmann G. Factors determining length of stay of surgical day-case patients. *Eur J Anaesthesiol.* 2001;18:314-21.

[119] Marshall SI, Chung F. Discharge criteria and complications after ambulatory surgery. *Anesth Analg.* 1999;88:508-17.

[120] Golembiewski J, Chernin E, Chopra T. Prevention and treatment of postoperative nausea and vomiting. *Am J Health Syst Pharm.* 2005;62:1247-60.

[121] Apfel CC, Laara E, Koivuranta M, Greim CA, Roewer N. A simplified risk score for predicting postoperative nausea and vomiting: conclusions from cross-validations between two centers. *Anesthesiology.* 1999;91:693-700.

[122] Watcha MF, White PF. Post-operative nausea and vomiting: its etiology, treatment and prevention. *Anesthesiology.* 1992;77:162-84.

[123] Apfel CC, Kranke P, Eberhart LH, Roos A, Roewer N. Comparison of predictive models for postoperative nausea and vomiting. *Br J Anaesth.* 2002;88:234-40.

[124] Koivuranta M, Laara E, Snare L, Alahuhta S. A survey of postoperative nausea and vomiting. *Anaesthesia.* 1997;52:443-9.

[125] Chinnappa V, Chung F. Postdischarge nausea and vomiting: an overlooked aspect of ambulatory anesthesia? *Can J Anaesth.* 2008;55:565-71.

[126] Yogendran S, Asokumar B, Cheng DC, Chung F. A prospective randomized double-blinded study of the effect of intravenous fluid therapy on adverse outcomes on outpatient surgery. *Anesth Analg.* 1995;80:682-6.

[127] Apfel CC, Korttila K, Abdalla M, Kerger H, Turan A, Vedder I, Zernak C, Danner K, Jokela R, Pocock SJ, Trenkler S, Kredel M, Biedler A, Sessler DI, Roewer N. A factorial trial of six interventions for the prevention of postoperative nausea and vomiting. *N Engl J Med.* 2004;350:2441-51.

[128] Elvir-Lazo OL, White PF. The role of multimodal analgesia in pain management after ambulatory surgery. *Curr Opin Anaesthesiol.* 2010;28:697-703.

[129] White PF. The role of non-opioid analgesic techniques in the management of pain after ambulatory surgery. *Anesth Analg.* 2002;94:577-85.

[130] Apfel CC, Kranke P, Katz MH, Goepfert C, Papenfuss T, Rauch S, Heineck R, Greim CA, Roewer N. Volatile anaesthetics may be the main cause of early but not delayed postoperative vomiting: a randomized controlled trial of factorial design. *Br J Anaesth.* 2002;88:659-68.

[131] Leslie K, Myles PS, Chan MT, Paech MJ, Peyton P, Forbes A, McKenzie D. ENIGMA Trial group. Risk factors for severe postoperative nausea and vomiting in a randomized trial of nitrous oxide-based vs nitrous oxide-free anaesthesia. *Br J Anaesth.* 2008;101:498-505.

[132] Le TP, Gan TJ. Update on the management of postoperative nausea and vomiting and postdischarge nausea and vomiting in ambulatory surgery. *Anesthesiol Clin.* 2010;28:225-49.

[133] White PF, Wang B, Tang J, Wender RH, Naruse R, Sloninsky A. The effect of intraoperative use of esmolol and nicardipine on recovery after ambulatory surgery. *Anesth Analg.* 2003;97:1633-8.

[134] Bell RF, Dahl JB, Moore RA, Kalso E. Peri-operative ketamine for acute post-operative pain: a quantitative and qualitative systematic review (Cochrane review). *Acta Anaesthesiol Scand.* 2005;49:1405-28.

[135] Keyes M. Management of postoperative nausea and vomiting in ambulatory surgery: the big little problem. *Clin Plast Surg.* 2013;40:447-52.

[136] Gan TJ, Meyer T, Apfel CC, Chung F, Davis PJ, Habib AS, Hooper VD, Kovac AL, Kranke P, Myles P, Philip BK, Samsa G, Sessler DI, Temo J, Tramèr MR, Vander Kolk C, Watcha M. Society for ambulatory anesthesia guidelines for the management of postoperative nausea and vomiting. *Anesth Analg.* 2007;105:1615-28.

[137] Elhakim M, Nafie M, Mahmoud K, Atef A. Dexamethasone 8 mg in combination with ondansetron 4 mg appears to be the optimal dose for the prevention of nausea and vomiting after laparoscopic cholecystectomy. *Can J Anaesth.* 2002;49:922-6.

[138] Mc Kenzie R, Lim Uy NT, Riley TJ, Hamilton DL. Droperidol/ ondansetron combination controls nausea and vomiting after tubal banding. *Anesth Analg.* 1996; 83:1218-22.

[139] Grimsehl K, Whiteside JB, MacKenzie N. Comparison of cyclizine and ondansetron for the prevention of postoperative nausea and vomiting in laparoscopic day-case gynaecological surgery. *Anaesthesia.* 2002; 57:61-5.

[140] Rawal N. Analgesia for day-case surgery. *Br J Anaesth.* 2001;87:73-87.

[141] Pavlin JD, Kent CD. Recovery after ambulatory anesthesia. *Curr Opin Anaesthesiol.* 2008;21:729-35.

[142] Claxton AR, McGuire G, Chung F, Cruise C. Evaluation of morphine versus fentanyl for postoperative analgesia after ambulatory surgical procedures. *Anesth Analg.* 1997;84:509-14.

[143] Awad IT, Chung F. Factors affecting recovery and discharge following ambulatory surgery. *Can J Anaesth.* 2006;53:858-72.

[144] Higgins PP, Chung F, Mezei G. Postoperative sore throat after ambulatory surgery. *Br J Anaesth.* 2002;88:582-4.

In: Advances in Surgical Procedures
Editor: Miriam Figueroa
ISBN: 978-1-63482-461-3

Chapter 2

New Materials and Techniques in General and Digestive Ambulatory Surgery

J. M. Suárez Grau, MD[1,2], S. García Ruiz, MD[2], C. Mendez García, MD[3], C. Rubio Chaves[4] and F. Docobo Durántez, Professor[4]
[1]General Hospital of Riotinto, Huelva, Spain
[2]Clinic Quirón Bilbao and Sagrado Corazón Seville, Spain
[3]University Hospital of Jerez, Spain
[4]University Hospital Virgen del Rocío, Seville, Spain

Abstract

Ambulatory surgery is constantly being updated, and is becoming more numerous interventions in this one day regime.

New materials and technological advances will certainly provide a large field of advantages for further proceedings in regimen of short-stay surgery.

New materials:

– Active Sutures: able to release substances at the site where they are applied. For example you sutures with antibiotics.

- Barbed Sutures (self-fixation): no need knotting, facilitating surgery and reducing surgical time.
- Self-gripping Meshes: no need of sutures or glues. This mesh improves the pain results. It reduces the surgical time.
- Biological synthetics meshes: usefull in hernia repair and in perianal fistulae.
- Laser: useful in hemorrhoids and perianal fistulae.

New techniques:

- Laparoscopy and Open surgery in inguinal hernia repair: TEP, TAPP, using new meshes and barbed sutures, traumatic (absorbable and metallic tackers) and non-traumatic fixation (glues);
- Hernioplasty using new meshes: self-gripping, biological meshes;
- Proctology interventions with laser: FILAC, HELP, LHP

All these advances in the surgery field, could improves the results in the ambulatory surgery in our centers. The main reasons are: minor surgical time, the rate of pain is very low, the discharge is in 6-8 hours after the intervention, the quick recovery and functional capacity to work, and the big satisfaction of the patients with these techniques.

Keywords: Ambulatory, surgery, materials, devices, innovations, sutures, mesh, laparoscopy

New Materials

1) Active Sutures

The sutures are the ones who have advanced in recent years, as the research focuses on finding new components that allow better absorption, less foreign body reaction and better integration with tissue. In addition to the synthesis of new products for sutures, they are trying to improve existing ones by adding substances to provide more resistance to the sutures.

It was well known to add antimicrobials such as triclosan to absorbable sutures polymer to increase the strength of sutures to infections. These active sutures prevented bacterial colonization and healing favored in an antiseptic environment. However, being described microbial resistance to triclosan, which new antiseptics are being investigated for covering sutures, such as chlorhexidine or short chain fatty acids. Both have proven effective in vitro for inhibition of bacterial growth and are harmless under biological conditions.

The short chain fatty acids are harmless substances used as preservatives in food and cosmetics. Their presence inhibits bacterial growth by creating a hostile environment for reproduction, yet is harmless to the native cell growth. Its low cost and absence of complications make it an ideal for creating active sutures to combat infection item.

Besides the addition of substances, it is improving in creating surfaces that hinder the development of infections. The discoveries of the ability of biofilm formation by pathogenic bacteria increased aggressiveness have put us on track for infection prevention can be done by preventing the formation of biofilm.

The last line of research is based on generating changes in the molecular structure of sutures to prevent bacterial growth. Nanotechnology, continuous development in other areas such as aerospace engineering or tele-communications, is allowing the appearance of materials that change under certain physiological conditions, resulting in a nano-porous structure With high surface area for protein binding. Then biologically active molecules are bound to the surface of the suture for subsequent release in vivo. Protein binding can be Achieved Rapidly in the operating room, and the process can be ready to enable the incorporation of a wide range of other therapeutic molecules.

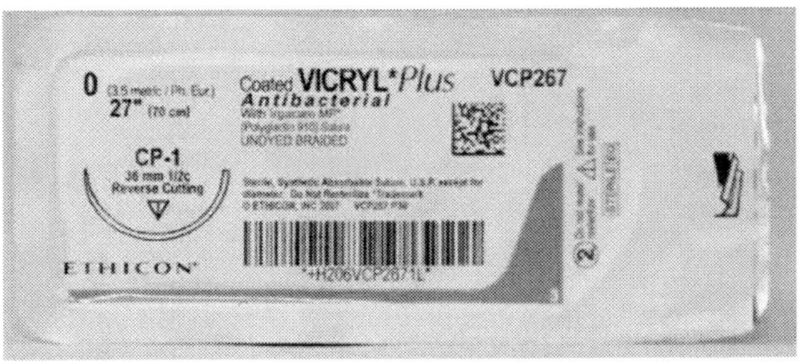

Active antibacterial suture: Vicryl Plus.

2) Self-Adhesions Sutures

The suture materials have been evolving throughout the years so that at the present time we have great amount of non-absorbable synthetic sutures as much absorbable, these last biopolymers with different times from absorption according to each necessity, as well as elastic sutures, impregnated in antiseptic substances, sutures that incorporate needles less and less traumatic and more and more and resistant... etc... in this epigraph we make mention to a special type of suture threads, the bearded sutures whose three-dimensional conformation presents a species of teeth or beards throughout its route (Figure 1) that once applied to the weave leaves the suture anchored preventing that the thread moves. Of this form they obtain that the approach of the edges is perfect and mainly, the benefit that seem to contribute is that they distribute the tension of the suture to length of all its extension.

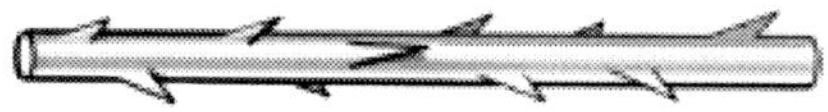

Schedule of bearded suture.

This bearded self-fixing system allowing the suture material for tissue approximation, which eliminates a long and tedious step in wound closure, the making of knots to attach and secure the connection.

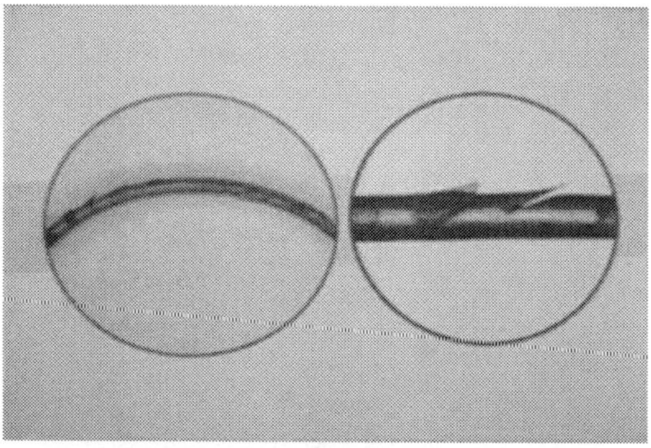

The helically barbs distributes tension across the entire length of the wound or tissue being approximated and eliminate the need for interrupted suture or tying knots. In this way some new opportunities appears above all in that cases of stitches are more difficult allowing surgeons to do things they could previously not do with traditional sutures, and, undoubtedly, making operating time shorter.

There are two main brands of bearded suture nowadays in the market: Quill ™ Knotless Tissue-Closure Device and V-Loc ™ Wound Closure Device.

- Quill ™ Knotless Tissue-Closure Device represents a revolutionary technology in wound closure made possible by bidirectional fixation within the wound. Its patented design

The Quill™ device is available in sizes 4/0 to 2. The bidirectional Quill ™ device is available in absorbable and non-absorbable materials and configurations including Monoderm ™, PDO, Nylon and Polypropylene. The unidirectional Quill ™ loop device is available in absorbable Monoderm ™ and PDO configurations.

- V-Loc ™ Wound Closure Device: it incorporates a double angle to the line marked by the base of the suture and the beard that, theoretically contributes takes more trustworthy and lasting anchorage.

The different types from sutures Pad ™ are mentioned in the following table:

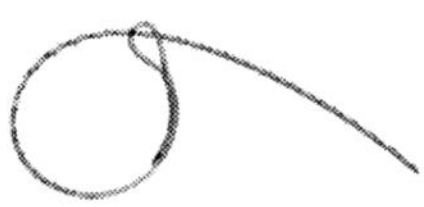

V-Loc (incorporate an eyelet to toughen the suture).

	V-Loc™ 90 device	V-Loc™ 180 device	V-Loc™ PBT Non-Absorbable Wound Closure Device
Tensile Strength	7 days, 90%; 14 days, 75%	7 days, 80%; 14 days, 75%; 21 days, 65%	Permanent
Absorption Profile	90-110 days	180 days	Permanent
Procedural Applications	Soft tissue approximation where support is required consistent with the absorption profile	Soft tissue approximation where support is required consistent with the absorption profile	Soft tissue approximation
Color	Undyed, violet	Clear, green	Blue
Composition	Glycolide, dioxanone and trimethylene carbonate	Copolymer of glycolic acid and trimethylene carbonate	Polybutester

3) Self-Gripping Meshes

In the last years we are attending to the birth of new prothesis devices for surgical treatment of abdominal wall pathology, that incorporate some measures like a three-dimensional conformation and a combination of biomaterials that confer an auto-adhesion capacity to them that makes unnecessary the use of fixation methods added.

They are in his majority, prothesis composed, elaborated from a base of polypropylene or polyester, both materials whose effectiveness is very well verified, and a biopolymer which is the one that support, of a way or another one, the anchorage capacity, without necessity to fix the prothesis with metallic tackers, stitches or biological glues, this reduces costs, operating time and risk of grabbing the nerve, with the consequent effect on the diminution of the postoperative pain.

In this sense, the mesh *Adhesix®, (Laboratoires Cousin Biotech, Wervicq Sud, France)* one is made up of a layer of polypropylene and on her a mixture of two biopolymers, polyethylene glycol (PEG) and polyvinylpyrrolidone (PVP) that to the contact with the humidity and the corporal heat forms an hydrogel with adherent characteristics, the mesh has not adhesiveness in dry environment.

Equally, the mesh *Hi-Tex Contact®, (Laboratoires Bioser, Montpellier, France)* made from a polyester base impregnated with alifatic polyurethane as a rough appendix is provided of a porous structure in 3D it accelerates its integration and colonization by the fibroblasts.

The Mesh *Parietene ™ Progrip ™ (Sofradim, Group Covidien® Trévoux, France)* is a partially absorbable mesh, of low molecular weight, composed of polypropylene monofilament and Polylactic Acid, this last as a shape of hooks which are inserted between the muscle fibers, allowing secure attachment from its inner surface, with less risk of mobilization of the hernia sac under the prosthesis.

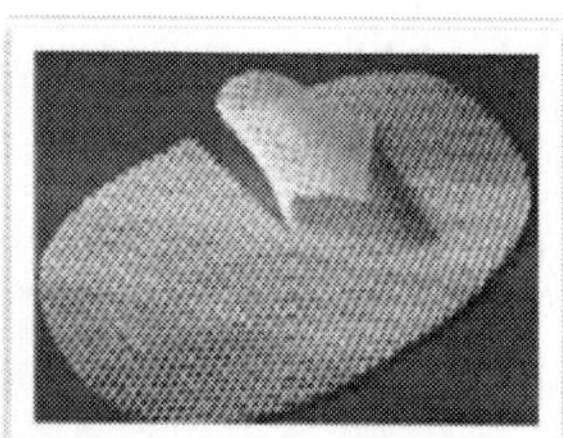
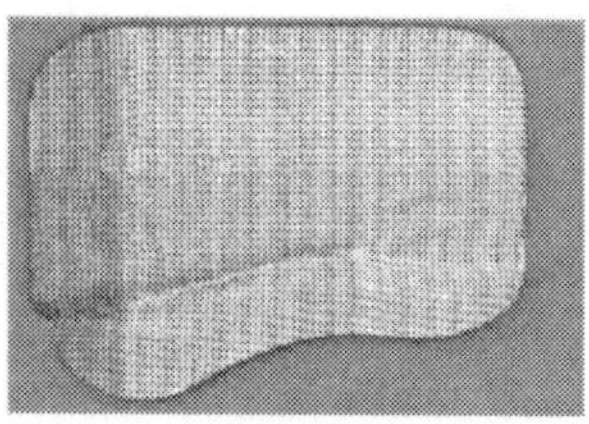

Progrip Mesh (self gripping mesh) in open surgery and for Laparoscopic Surgery.

4) Biological-Synthetics Meshes: Hernia Repair and in Perianal Fistulae

Hernia Repair

Biologic mesh development resulted from a search for a biomaterial that could address the problems associated with permanent synthetic mesh, including chronic inflammation and foreign body reaction, stiffness and fibrosis, and mesh infection. New biological or synthetics absorbable meshes can be use in ambulatory surgery in order to decrease the pain, surgical time and infection associated with the surgery procedure.

Hernia Plug BIO-A polymer (Gore Bio-A; W. L. Gore and Associates, Flagstaff, Ariz): Hernia Plug is a porous fibrous structure composed of synthetic copolymer that is bioabsorbed in approximately six months. It is both biocompatible and nonantigenic. The GORE® BIO-A® Hernia Plug repairs hernia defects by promoting a well-organized tissue response, while markedly reducing chronic complications associated with permanent implants. The unique design of the plug serves as a scaffold to facilitate tissue generation, and is highly adaptable and easily tailored to create an optimal fit for the defect. Results in an experience multicentric for two years of follow-up show the GORE Bioabsorbable Hernia Plug with onlay mesh is effective with minimal short-term complications (3.6%) and minimal long-term pain (3% incidence of pain at two years).

Biologic Meshes: Given the high cost of most of these materials and the limited available data, biologic mesh should be used judiciously and only when permanent synthetic mesh is inappropriate, such as in the contaminated field.

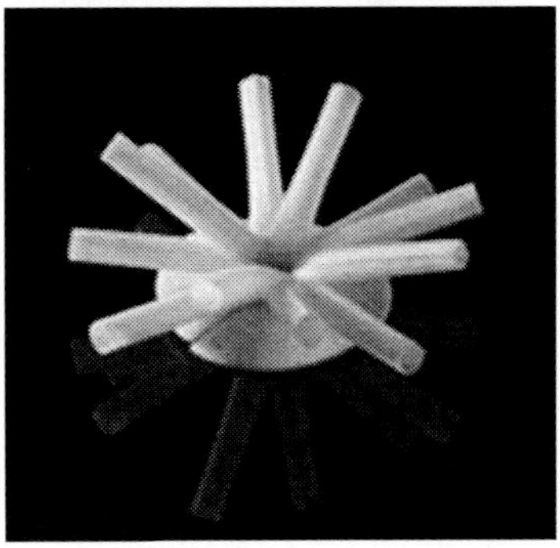

Gore BioA- Inguinal Hernia Plug..

Fistulae Repair

The anal fistula plug is a noncutting, sphincter-sparing technique. It has low morbidity and can be repeated if necessary. We can use this procedure in patients who has had prior drainage with a seton before placement of the plug. The anal fistula Plugs are in this moment: 1)treated porcine submucosa (Cook Biodesign; Cook Medical, Bloomington, Ind) 2) synthetic bioabsorbable polymer (Gore Bio-A; W. L. Gore and Associates, Flagstaff, Ariz)

The fistula tract should be curetted, and the external opening débrided deeply. The plug should be advanced in one direction (inside to outside)from the internal opening to the external opening. The base of the plug is seated at the internal opening. We sutured the base to the internal opening with absorbable suture to close the internal opening over the plug. The excess plug at the external opening is removed with shears, and the external opening left open (such a natural drainage). Success rates have been reported in a range from 43% to 87%. In our experience, around the 50% of the patients had good results with total resolution of the fistula.

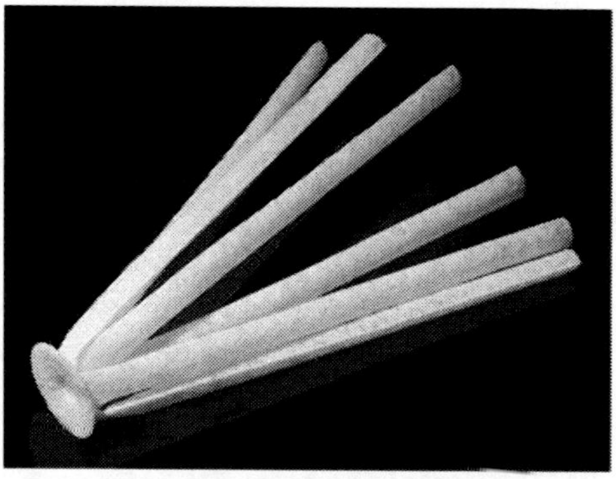

Fistuale Plug Bio-A.

5) Laser in Proctology Procedures

Ambulatory surgery is in a constant development because, by its nature, requires that operating times are reduced and recovery occurs most easily, without postoperative complications and without hospital cares for the patient. In this sense, any innovation to perform safe surgery in less time and with a rapid recovery, is particularly susceptible to being included in outpatient surgery programs.

In proctology, the increased difficulty in performing ambulatory techniques is postoperative pain, since it is an extremely sensitive area. Most proctologic interventions also include a complete removal of tissue, which greatly increases the discomfort during recovery. In this sense, the use of proctologic laser allows first performing an occlusion to treat the pathology without removing it.

The laser proceeds very selectively to the lesion, minimally damaging adjacent tissues. It produces minimal tissue damage, so pain is drastically reduced or it even completely disappears after surgery. So has fewer side effects needless destruction of healthy tissue and inflammation.

Laser devices used in proctology are made of glass fiber optic, transmitting the pulse of laser light right in the area you need. Its minimum size prevents extensive manipulations on the surrounding tissues, allowing addressing areas inaccessible to conventional surgery, with greater assurance of results. The console device allows you to adjust the dose of energy transmitted in each incision and in total intervention, so that the desired results are calibrated exactly. The laser also produces the sealing of nerve terminals that conduct the sensation of pain, by which the patient suffers at all during the procedure.

The procedure is ambulatory and requires a minimum hospital stay, blood loss and anesthesia needed is reduced. After surgery, the individual who has gone through she should just stay a couple of hours in the hospital before going home.

The fiber system used is different according to the pathology. For perianal fistula is required of an optical fiber blunt and flexible, that does not generate false paths during surgery. To address an intermittent pulse laser and prolonged periodic moderate frequency. The fiber should be blunt to produce a circumferential burn to close the fistula tract and promotes the healing thereof, since the objective of this intervention is the sealing of the duct and eliminate chronic granulation tissue which remains active infection.

For the treatment of hemorrhoids, an optical fiber with change angular tip, higher precision is used and is capable of moving as a needle, with minimal trauma, within solid tissue. The laser pulse used should be intermittent, short period, with high frequency and high energy. These high-energy short pulses allow vascular occlusion by the hemorrhoid vessels blood clotting inside, with a solid seal that prevents vessel patency. If the pulses were of long duration, the heat transfer to the surroundings of the vessel could cause a painful and burn recovery worse.

New Techniques

1) Inguinal Hernia Repair

Surgical pathology of abdominal wall is one of the most frequent pathology operated by ambulatory surgery system.

Traditionally, main issue that surgeons keeping in mind had been the hernia relapse. A long time ago, this concern is relatively well managed, because of the new prothesis made of different biomaterials and tridimensional conformations which get a free-tension repair.

Once this objective could be considered obtained, the interest of surgical community all over the world has been deposited in other clinical aspects of quality assistance. For this reason, the most of actual researches are going deeply in new techniques that besides of being safe and effective could provide the maximum comfort, with less postoperative pain, in an efficient way from an economic point of view.

In that sense, new methods of fixation, self-fixation prosthesis and minimal invasive surgery play an important role.

a) Inguinal Hernioplasty Without Sutures

The new availability of prosthetics and biomaterials has allowed to invent ever more anatomical surgical repair techniques and concurrently, the fact of eliminating, or at least reducing, the need of additional fixation has had a big impact in improving the efficiency of major outpatient surgery units: on the one hand making shorter operative times in order to optimizing the operating room occupation, and on the other hand, minimizing the risk of nerve damage, reducing in that way the chances of postoperative pain, essential issue in cases where discharges of patients have to be established at an early stage.

Fixation with biological glues

We have disposable two kinds of biomaterials derivatives of cyanoacrylate and fibrin sealants.

The cyanocrylate have shown a high adhesive capacity with minimal inflammatory response, which added to the simplicity of management, its low cost and its so-called antibacterial properties, placed it at the head of the biological glues used for the fixation of prostheses in hernia surgery. They do not require a special conservation or a complex processing. Its mode of employment is limited to pour a few drops of product in strategic places where traditional suture stitches would be situated and allow to dry for few seconds.

Fibrin sealants are chemical compounds containing among other products: fibrinogen, fibronectin, factor XIII, and as VEGF, TGF-B, EGF and FGF growth factors. They produce a fibroblastic proliferation in the first moments after the placement of the mesh, which helps correct integration and an optimal final result. It has a cost significantly higher than the previous, and processing prior to their use which requires a deep knowledge of the product. In the case of heterologous fibrin sealants *(Tissucol®)* this means a correct conservation in cold, removing several minutes before use and follow the instructions in the commercial kit that involves a transfer of product to different syringes and continuous agitation. Its application above the mesh is not done directly, but through a propeller device that sprayed product.

In the case of autologous fibrin sealants *(Vivostat®)* the cost is even higher. This system involves the removal of a sample of blood from the patient, prior to surgery and its treatment in a special container that extracted from the patient's own fibrin. Its main advantage is the elimination of possible immunological reactions.

Self fixating Prosthesis

Self fixating meshes more utilized in One–day surgery are the previously commented, Adhesix® and Parietene™ Progrip™.

The mesh Parietene™ Progrip™ (Covidien®) appears in three modalities, two of them of elliptical form, specially designed to adapt to the anatomy of the inguinal region, with an adjustable auto-adhesive lapel around the cord, either towards the left, or towards right. The third variant is a flat plate of 15x9 cm2.

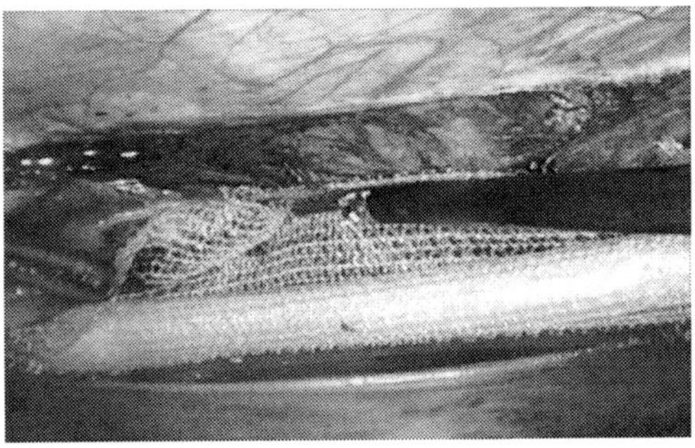

Progrip in Laparoscopic TAPP.

It's easy to use, surgeons only have to complete the dissection of the anatomical area and put the mesh in correct orientation, making sure the spermatic cord is suitably rounded by the lapel, once done this, last step is make a soft pressure pushing down for a few seconds in order to PLA grips taking place on the surface. After that, only rest closing muscular fascia, cellular subcutaneous tissue and skin above it.

Adhesix® mesh has four varieties about size and shape: one oval shape, and three specially designed for inguinal region, one of them completely plate and the other two types with an aperture for the spermatic cord placement.

Its use is similar to the one before described for Progrip®, but in this case the adhesiveness of the mesh depends in great measure of the humidity of the surface. It is so important checking the correct position of the mesh before starting the closure for avoiding undesirable movements of it.

b) Laparoscopy Surgery in Inguinal Hernia Repair: TEP, TAPP

The advantages of this method include less pain, smaller scars, and an ability to visualize both sides of the abdomen through a single approach. That being said, this is the preferred technique when there are hernias present on both sides. It is also preferred when a hernia has recurred following a prior repair, as the surgeon is able to dissect through non-scarred tissues in order to fix the defect.

The laparoscopic approach is ideal for patients who are obese, have recurrence from a prior open approach, have bilateral hernias, or require an operation that may result in a shorter convalescence (ambulatory surgery). All laparoscopic inguinal hernia repairs require placing mesh in the preperitoneal space to reinforce the myopectineal orifice. This was initially performed with a TAPP approach requiring initial entry into the abdominal cavity followed by division of the peritoneum and subsequent entry into the preperitoneal space. TAPP is preferred for patients with a large hernia or a prior infraumbilical abdominal incision because the contents of a large hernia can be assessed and reduced from the abdominal cavity, and scar tissue from a prior midline incision makes TEP entry more difficult due to adhesions.

TEP is the most cost-efficient technique in terms of outcome, and recovery/reinsertion in work. Although TEP is a demanding technique, with a longer learning curve than TAPP, the results in ambulatory surgery make it the most appropriate laparoscopic technique for a discharge on the same day (with high rates of security against TAPP, because there is no access to the intra-abdominal cavity).

Indications in the Table:

TEP versus TAPP		
Attributes	**TAPP**	**TEP**
Indications	Bilateral inguinal hernia	Bilateral inguinal hernia
	Recurrence from prior open inguinal hernia surgery with Mesh or TEP Surgery.	Reucurrence from prior open inguinal hernia surgery without Mesh.
	Prior Midline abdominal or preperitoneal surgery.	Smaller or normal unilateral hernia (fully reductible defect).
	Large, partially reductible hernias	
	Obese patient	
Common Complications	Bowel injury	Bleeding from injured epigastric vessels or corona mortis.
	Port site hernia	Incomplete hernia reduction
	Mesh exposure to bowel due to incomplete peritoneal closure or peritoneal tears (causing obstructions)	Small peritoneal tears (undetectable) with pneumoperitoneum (causing pain and avoiding ambulatory surgery)

2) Proctology Interventions with Laser

FILAC (FIstula LAser Closure)

The perianal fistula is mostly mild pathology of chronic tendency, so although most cases are not serious or present complications, the high recurrence rate and the difficulty of finding a definitive solution make it a condition that requires a careful treatment.

The usual treatment of perianal fistula has been performed in ambulatory surgical programs for years, because they are usually not painful or complicated treatments. Fistulotomy and traditional fistulectomy involve significant discomfort in the late postoperative period, because the healing of these wounds usually requires time, but not usually cause pain in the immediate postoperative period, since the effect of anesthesia adequately control these symptoms.

FILAC technique involves occlusion of the fistula energy emitted by a blunt laser fiber. The energy transmitted to the tissue inside the path causes scarring that is immediately after the emission of energy and which is produced by the coagulation of proteins usually granulation tissue filled the duct. For proper sealing, it is necessary to treat all abscesses that may exist and completely remove the remains of the fistulous tract infection. The recommended method to eliminate the infection is the placement of a drain placed between the internal and the external fistulous opening fistula orifice to cease issuing pus. This drain help us following placement of the fiber laser through the hole.

When the path is clean, you can proceed to sealing by laser, to be held from the internal fistula opening retreating toward the outer and never backwards, to prevent the formation of abscessed cavity and false ways to annul the effect of occlusion. If the internal fistulous chronic signs of granulation, the production of a small mucosal flap to reinforce the effect of the laser on the mucosa is recommended.

The laser pulses must be programmed into the device to be moderate, intermittent frequency and maintained timing. Fiber is slowly removed from inner hub to the outer, we left the checking successively closed by a soft tip reintroduction fiber path.

In the external fistulous opening any action may not be necessary, although some authors recommend excision circumferential external fistulous opening with monopolar scalpel, favoring the creation of a stronger and without chronic granulation tissue scar. The removal of surrounding tissue has not been shown to cause better results, but a slight increase postoperative pain, so it is only recommended in patients with fistulas very long evolution in which the external fistulous opening is large.

The FILAC has no contraindication size of the fistula or by location, since not require excision of tissue damage or cross brings many fewer complications than other more aggressive techniques. Can be used in e intersphinterics extrasphinterics fistulas, provided the path is well defined.

The main limitation of this technique are multiple perianal fistulas involving the difficulty in occluding fistulas branched, especially if you have not managed to track properly. In these cases, you can make partial occlusions localized paths to progressively decrease the size of the fistula and the roads that form, to meet with a single journey.

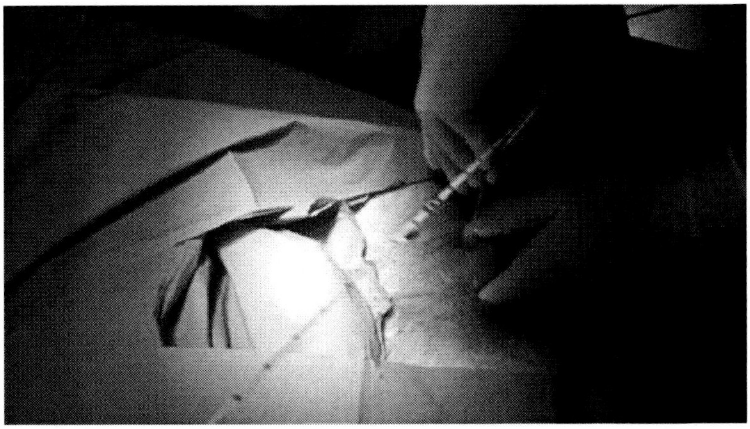

FILAC: in an extrasphinteric anal fistulae.

LHP

Venous occlusion hemorrhoid laser is effective for the treatment of this disease that prevents the main postoperative complication option: the pain of excision of tissue. In performing this technique, the hemorrhoidal package is not removed, leaving a wound, but it is coagulated and occluded under the mucosa as a solid callus prevents venous dilatation and consequent hemorrhoidal prolapse.

By leaving scar tissue included under the mucosa, is not indicated in patients with grade IV hemorrhoids bulky, since the excess tissue of these patients makes their removal is necessary to obtain a satisfactory result. The best indication of hemorrhoidal laser occlusion are patients with grade II-III hemorrhoids, especially those who have presented episodes of rectal bleeding not associated with prolapse or those who complain of pruritus ani.

The technique is performed in the operating room under general or spinal anesthesia, as it requires an anal dilation anuscope that allows control the process of hemorrhoidal occlusion. You can place the patient in a position to Seville knife or lithotomy. Postoperative not exceed the length of anesthetic recovery as surgical discomfort is minimal.

To occlusion, three or four small incisions are made in the base of each hemorrhoid pedicle going to try (usually in the anterior pedicle right, rear right and left side). These incisions are made in the mucocutaneous junction, on the anoderm, before you begin to glimpse the hemorrhoidal package. It is not necessary that the incisions maximum of 2 mm in length, and we only need the caliber of the laser fiber. The fiber should be introduced parallel to the anal canal, without going through the anal mucosa to prevent bleeding and even exceed the length of the hemorrhoidal plexus. From that point, the laser pulses which have previously been programmed into the console to be short, high-energy start.

The laser pulses are applied repetitively removing the fiber over the hemorrhoidal package and through the anoscope watching a hemorrhoid lie clotting integrity of the anal mucosa and the internal anal sphincter is maintained is performed.

If the technique is performed well, after occlusion must observe a discrete skin retraction anus into the anal canal and the absence of bleeding through surgical wounds. If you notice any bleeding, can coagulate using long laser pulses, assuming the burn could cause pain.

After recovery from anesthesia, the patient can be discharged. The most frequent postoperative discomfort usually appear after 48 hours after surgery, when the occlusion is more established and has triggered inflammatory response in the area.

Long term results are unknown for this technique and the real rate of recurrence as well. Detractors argue that the results are poor, considering that hemorrhoids treated are in moderate degrees, they should have final results regardless of the treatment applied. The reality is that no treatment has been shown definitively described to eradicate hemorrhoids, you always have a recurrence rate, and laser results has been no worse than other painful techniques.

HeLP

Besides hemorrhoidal vein occlusion we have described, the laser can be used to generate a selective hemorrhoidal artery occlusion, which devascularice hemorrhoids by cutting the blood flow. By high energy pulses coagulation arterial dilation hemorrhoidal limiting is achieved. It can be used as the sole method or associated with LHP.

To perform this technique, you must first locate the artery going to flirt. Devices that are marketed include ecodoppler system coupled to Anoscope to find the arterial pulse before I coagulate. The administration of laser energy will also be incorporated into the anoscope, which is much simpler power management at the required point.

It is important to locate 3-4 hemorrhoidal arteries occlude want because if the treatment is performed in part, recurrence is more likely to be a fine vascular network connected to each other. Given the difficulty of finding all packages (in patients with previous vascular problems, for example), a LHP proccedure associated is a simple technique that does not require selective localization of blood vessels.

The recovery is in 3-4 hours after intervention, with no pain and major complications in follow-up. Total recovery (work and normal life) is usually complete within 24 hours.

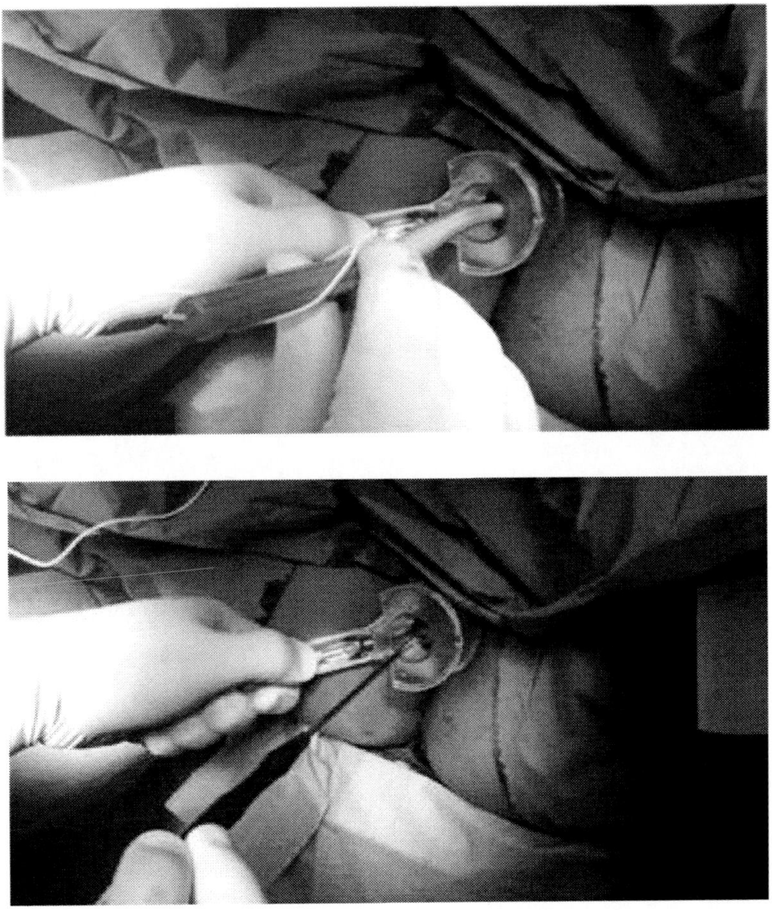

Doppler detection of hemorroidals artery and Devacularization with Laser.

In: Advances in Surgical Procedures
Editor: Miriam Figueroa
ISBN: 978-1-63482-461-3

Chapter 3

Ambulatory Surgery in Orthopaedics: Prevalence, Complications and Long-Term Outcomes

***Omar Faour Martín*[1*] *and Miguel Ángel Martín Ferrero*[2]**
[1]Service of Traumatology and Orthopaedic Surgery,
Hospital of Ávila- Sacyl, Spain
[2]Service of Traumatology and Orthopaedic Surgery,
Clinic Universitary Hospital of Valladolid, Spain

Abstract

The concept of day surgery is becoming an increasingly important part of elective surgery worldwide. Relentless pressures to cut costs may constrain clinical judgments regarding the most appropriate location for a patient's surgical care. Ambulatory surgery in Orthopaedics has shown in our institution to be able to provide good-quality service. There still seems to be potential to increase the proportion of these procedures. Therefore, surgeons and anaesthesiologists must strongly adhere to strict patient selection criteria in order to reduce complications in the immediate postoperative term. We expose a revision of more than 10.000

[*] Contact person: O. Faour Martín. Email: ofmartin@msn.com

patients during the last twenty years following the protocols of our Ambulatory Surgery Unit. Major complications recorded in our revision were minimal without any mortal case. Unplanned overnight admission rate of 0.14% was achieved and a high rate of ambulatory substitution in procedures studied was registered.

Keywords: Ambulatory, orthopaedics, surgery, procedures

1. Introduction

Orthopaedic surgery is the branch of surgery concerned with conditions involving the musculoskeletal system. In recent years, the prevalence of musculoskeletal procedures has drastically increased around the world. In this context, the notion of day surgery is becoming an increasingly important part of elective surgery worldwide [1]. Decreased healthcare costs, efficacy of operative care, patient's satisfaction, and dedicated staff are important factors that have led to an increase in its popularity.

Public health policies have promoted ambulatory surgery. This has been one of the most important and dynamic changes in medical care during the last decades. Many managers consider it as a way to increase and enhance access and control costs [2]. At this respect, it has been estimated that the costs for day-surgery procedures are 25–68% lower compared with inpatient care [3,4].

However, this large diffusion has occurred without the outcome assessments that are usually associated with such an important change in health care practices and policies [5]. The potential advantages of day-surgery practice disappear when patients require emergency care due to adverse events. In this respect, the data provided by Matilla et al. [6], after a thorough study of day surgery of all specialties in Finland, revealed rates of admission of 5.9% and readmission within 24 hours postoperatively of 0.1%. In other studies, unplanned admissions after ambulatory surgery were thought to occur in approximately 0.5% to 1.5% of cases [7,8]. Direct admissions from a day surgical unit during a five-year study [9] varied by service: 0.80% for gynecologic, 0.79% for orthopaedic and 0.57% for general surgery departments. The main reported risk factors for hospital admission were duration of the surgical procedure, general anesthesia, bleeding and uncontrolled pain.

2. Our Experience in Orthopaedics Day-Surgery

In many centers, ambulatory procedures are considered the norm for programmed surgical treatments. Local structural and functional differences may explain the variation in outpatient surgery activity still seen between hospitals together with different patient and procedure-related selection criteria [10].

We have performed an updated of data registered previously of our experience in orthopaedic day surgery [11]. The centre is a teaching university hospital with a referral population of up to 300,000 people. It belongs to the National Health System, which provides free universal coverage and is financed through the resources of the Spanish Public Administration. The Orthopedic Academic Department has an Ambulatory Surgery Unit, composed of three consultants with independent functionality. Four to six surgical sessions are held each week. The upgrade comprises the incorporation of recent years so that the data of patients operated in this regime from June 1993 to november 2014 are collected.

Inclusion Criteria for Orthopaedic Day-Surgery

As in the previous years, the patient inclusion criteria for orthopaedic ambulatory surgery in our institution are considered as follows [12]:

a) Patient comorbidities: the patients could not have any uncontrolled metabolic or psychiatric illness, drug addiction, coagulopathy, epilepsy, history of severe anesthetic complications, symptomatic cardiac disease six months previous to surgery, body mass index exceeding 30, or be undergoing anticoagulant treatment. We considered patients that were I and II or controlled III and IV status, according to the preoperative risk criteria established by the American Society of Anesthesiologists (ASA). Controlled arterial hypertension, stable chronic obstructive pulmonary disease and diabetes treated with oral agents were not considered as exclusion criteria.
b) Social status of the patient: the patient needed an adequate family environment with an available telephone, no architectural obstacles, a responsible caregiver for the 24-48 hour postoperative period, easy

land communication with a hospital, and needed to be over 18 months of age.

c) Surgical technique: patients with no complex preoperative preparation, with little bleeding and mild physiological aggression were included. The postoperative period should have been managed without invasive procedures.

d) Anesthesia: possibility of using a safe method that allowed for a fast recovery profile.

Discharge after Ambulatory Orthopaedic Surgery

Patients were discharged according to Korttila´s criteria for day surgery [13]:

- Vital signs stable for at least 1 hour.
- Patient oriented to person, place, and time
- Able to tolerate orally administered fluids
- Able to void, to dress and to walk without assistance
- No more than minimal nausea or vomiting
- Absence of excessive pain and bleeding
- The patient must be discharged by both anesthetist and surgeon
- Written instructions for the postoperative period at home, including a contact place and a person who may be telephoned, need to be reinforced; presence of a responsible adult to escort patient.

The patient had to be able to swallow and cough as well, and explicit consent from the patient or the adult caregiver was necessary for discharge.

Preoperative and Immediate Postoperative Management

The day before surgery all patients were personally given detailed oral and written instructions to follow for the ambulatory procedure. Hospital contact phone numbers for any eventuality were given.

During the immediate postoperative period, patients were transferred to a recovery room and discharged whenever they met the criteria described above. In most of the cases, all drainages (if placed) were removed the day after the surgical procedure.

Checks were done by a home-hospital unit during the first 48 hours after discharge. This unit used a public phone to ask all the questions about the process. All patients were reviewed in the surgeon's office within 7 days of discharge.

A clinical evaluation, both in the preoperative period and one week after surgery, was performed using the SF36 questionnaire [14]. It contains 36 items in nine separate domains. Eight of these comprise two or more items and the final one has only one item. Each domain is computed to give a scaled score of 0-100. It was adapted for use in our country and is widely recommended as a tool for health status assessments in care settings [14]. Subjective satisfaction, scored from 0-10, was registered, as well as an actual comparative satisfaction study with a subgroup of patients operated on in an inpatient regime of the main processes. This latter group comprised patients operated on by orthopedic surgeons from our institution that work outside our ambulatory surgery unit. Patients that would not fulfill the inclusion criteria for outpatient surgery because of clinical reasons were excluded.

Updated Results

The sex distribution of the 11,355 patients evaluated was 4,326 males (38.2%) and 7029 females (61.8%). The mean age was 42.3 years (range 2-81). The age distribution was as follows: 69 patients younger than 15 years old (0.60%), 1,340 aged between 15 and 30 years (11.9%), 2135 between 30 to 45 years (18.7%), 3,997 between 45 and 60 years (35.1%), between 60 and 75 years 3213 (28.4%) and 601 patients (5.6%) over 75 years.

The number of patients that were living in rural areas was 1,851 (16.3%), compared to 9504 (83.7%) patients that inhabited urban areas.

ASA scores were distributed as follows: ASA I in 6132 cases (54.0%), ASA II in 4,962 cases (43.7%), ASA III in 261 cases (2.3%) and no patients with ASA IV.

Intervened diseases represented a wide range of pathologies: knee arthroscopy for meniscus resection, meniscus suture, and anterior cruciate ligament (ACL) reconstruction, shoulder arthroscopy for rotator cuff repair, acromioplasty and instability treatment joint mobilization, removal of osteosynthesis material, excision of synovial cysts, opening of pulleys for trigger fingers, tenotomies, removal of external fixators, arthrodesis and arthroplasty of the fingers, osteosynthesis of hand fractures, fasciectomy for Dupuytren´s disease, removal of foreign bodies, nerve decompression (carpal tunnel syndrome, Guyon's syndrome, cubital algoparesia in the elbow); excision of neuromas, amputation of fingers, correction of toe deformities (hallux valgus, hammer toes) fingernail operations, skin grafting, neurorrhaphy, nerve grafting, palliative surgery of peripheral nerve paralysis, tenorrhaphy and tenolysis.

Regional anesthesia was used in 8289 cases (73%), local anesthesia was used in 2,964 cases of (26.1%), and general anesthesia was used in 102 cases (0.9%).

The average time of the intraoperative period, from patient entry to the theater until exit to the recovery postsurgical area, was 28 minutes (range 10-117). The average time the patient spent in the unit, from arrival to discharge, was 184 minutes (range 24-322).

No major complications were recorded. Only 16 patients (0.14%) required overnight admission after surgery. The reasons for admission were suspected pneumothorax (two patients), lack of a responsible adult to accompany the patient (four patients), non-acceptance of discharge due to general discomfort (four patients), monitoring the vascular status of the toes where slow revascularization persisted two hours after surgery (four patients), and vomiting (four patients). The main characteristics of these 16 patients were: mean age of 70.4 years (range: 61-78); ASA grade III in 12 cases (75%) and grade II in four cases (25%); regional anesthesia had been administered in eight cases (50%) and general anesthesia in seven patients (42.9%). The mean surgical mean duration was 67 minutes (range 35-119).

59 patients (0.52%) left the hospital by ambulance due to the postoperative indication of not being able to bear weight on a lower limb. 147 patients needed attention at the emergency department during the first 24 hours after discharged (1.3%) because of pain (108 patients) or bleeding (39 patients), with four subsequent hospitalizations after shoulder arthroscopy, six because of knee pain and swelling after ACL reconstruction and one after arthroscopic knee arthrolysis.

During the first 48 hours after surgery, a medical consultation by phone was needed by 2124 patients (18.7%) due to discomfort (1020 patients), concerns regarding postoperative prescriptions (224 patients), or bleeding (880 patients). Most of these queries were sorted out by phone.

Painkillers were needed during a mean postoperative period of 5.2 days (range 1 -29). The following complications were recorded during the first clinical revision that took place seven days after surgery: superficial infections were found in seven patients, which resolved with outpatient care; a metacarpophalangeal prosthesis infection in a rheumatoid patient that required surgical revision; two deep infections in diabetic patients operated on for Dupuytren's disease, one of which needed amputation of the fifth finger; suture dehiscence in five patients, one of whom was diabetic; intra-articular hematoma due to suction drainage malfunction in seven patients. The number of patients requiring admission between postoperative 24 hours and 28 days after surgery was eight (0.06%).

Subjective outcomes made reference to those patients capable of understanding and answering the items of the SF-36 questionnaire (11299 patients, 99.5%). The results of the questionnaire revealed a significant improvement in the quality of life index in postoperative values as compared to the preoperative values ($p < 0.0001$), in all the items: *general health, limitation of activities, physical health problems, emotional health problems, social activities, pain, energy and emotions*

The mean satisfaction value for the management of all surgical procedures was of 8.64/10 (range 4-10). The results for satisfaction between in Day and inpatient surgery during the last five years did not show significant differences overall, so the ambulatory management of the procedure did not mean a decrease in patient satisfaction.

Quality Indicators

To sum up, our experience in Ambulatory Orthopedic Surgery has presented the following quality indicators:

- Unplanned overnight admission: 0.14%
- Readmission rate within 24 hours: 0.09%
- Readmission rate 1-28 days after discharge: 0.06%
- Emergency room visits rate: 1.3%
- Cancellation of booked procedures: 1.51%
- Ambulatory Orthopedic Surgery/All elective surgeries of the orthopedic department for the period studied: 39.2%.

Reasons of cancellation of booked procedures (164) were: acute illness in 114 cases (73.8%), decision by the patient in 18 cases (10.3%), and lack of surgical material in 32 cases (15.9%).

The substitution rate for different surgical interventions, defined as the number of ambulatory surgeries divided by all surgeries performed for a specific procedure [7], was as follows:

- *Carpal tunnel decompression: 97.2%*
- *Arthroscopic meniscectomy: 77,5%*
- *Acromioplasty/bursectomy:83.4%*
- *Hallux valgus correction:96.2%*
- *Rhizarthrosis surgery: 87.2%*
- *Osteosynthesis of hand and wrist bones: 87.3%*
- *Anterior cruciate ligament reconstruction: 36.4%*
- *Dupuytren disease:88.4%*
- *Arthroscopical Shoulder inestability repair: 42.7%*
- *Tenolysis of trigger fingers:98.9%*

The number of total ambulatory procedures without unplanned admission was of 11,320. The mean direct cost of day-admission in our institution during the last twenty years was of 375.4 Euros. The economic global results coming from the data registered in our revision indicate that the saving has been at least of 4, 2495,627 Euros.

3. Present and Future

The aim of our actualization was to determine the clinical and quality indicators of our experience in Orthopedic Day Surgery in a revision of more than 11,000 patients during the last twenty years, mainly in relation to the unplanned overnight admission and readmission rates. Also we consider that the description of the main characteristics of the patients that experimented complications and the patient comparative satisfaction rate between the ambulatory and non-ambulatory procedures is a fundamental issue. As such, our revision may provide a benchmark to evaluate future outpatient orthopedic surgery disposition rates. Clinical indicators from the SF-36 score revealed favorable outcomes in the immediate postoperative term. The results for satisfaction between in Day and inpatient surgery did not show significant differences, so the ambulatory management did not lead to a decrease in patient satisfaction.

Ambulatory surgery in Orthopedics has shown in our institution to be able to provide good-quality service, with high patient satisfaction. There still seems to be potential to increase the proportion of these procedures, and best practices should be sought. The efficacy and quality of the process itself requires further study. Figures for clinical indicators and the proportion of day surgery of all elective surgeries at individual hospitals, and nationally, should be made easily accessible for benchmarking and quality control with an automated reporting system. In future, day surgery should be the norm for elective surgery.

Assessment of quality of care is not only important for health control, but fundamental for the development of the expanding day-surgery service. Relentless pressures to cut costs and to provide services in the least costly setting may, in the absence of contrary evidence, constrain clinical judgments regarding the most appropriate location for a patient's surgical care [2].

Our patient selection criteria were rather uniform and in line with present-day recommendations [15]. In the future, the demand for day surgery in the increasing elderly population and in patients with notable comorbidities will undoubtedly increase. Therefore, surgeons and anesthesiologists must strongly adhere to those criteria in order to reduce complications in the immediate postoperative time [16]. Some of these risk factors may be proxies for surgical and/or case complexity; however, there is currently no generally accepted measure of procedure complexity.

Major complications in our review were minimal, and there were no deaths. Despite a controlled IV ASA risk was not considered as an exclusion criteria, no patient with this condition were registered due to a concomitant disease, such as coagulopathy or cardiopathy that excluded them from our study. Quality of care was measured by rates regarding with unplanned overnight admission, patient returns to hospital within 24 hours, admission within 24 hours and during the first month after surgery, and cancellation of booked procedures. Those outcomes have been lower than data shown by other studies about ambulatory surgery overall [16-19].

Efforts must be carrying out in the management of Ambulatory Surgery in Orthopedics in order to reduce the unplanned admission rates. In this way, a deep preoperative specific clinical evaluation must be performed closed in time to the intervention in order to detect conditions that contraindicate an ambulatory procedure. Operations must be performed as minimally invasive as possible and clear indications must be given to the patients during the first hours with a tight ambulatory follow-up.

As in other articles [17-19], pain and bleeding still continue being the most common reason of adverse events after ambulatory surgical procedures. In our experience, most of the patients needing unexpected overnight admission or readmission during the first 24 hours after surgery, presented an advanced age, ASA condition of III, or a considerable surgical duration.

In order to minimize complications in ambulatory surgery, we consider essential to act on factors influencing on immediate recovery, such as postoperative analgesia and anti-emetic prophylaxis [20]. In the same way, dressing of the limbs after surgery is critical. An inappropriate choice or placement could cause important and serious adverse events, and it is necessary to avoid bandages that could create compression and vascular problems, such as a full plaster.

In addition, we have recorded a high replacement rate for procedures such as knee arthroscopy, osteosynthesis of the hand, or carpal tunnel decompression, when compared with other published studies that report these rates up to 83.1%, 70.7%, and 64.3% respectively [21].

Ambulatory surgery in Orthopaedics may be consider a present and future essential part of the management of the specialty. Units Ambulatory Surgery have, within the National Health System as well as in the private sector, a considerable development over the past fifteen years That lead to an increasing efficiency in the care of patients eligible for orthopaedic surgical procedures that previously were admitted in conventional hospital units. The relative novelty of this healthcare modality, its important dissemination, the diversity of organizational, structural and functional configurations must be taken into account. Its significant impact in terms of quality and patient safety, make this kind of Unit, as one of the elements of priority in health politics. Standard criteria of quality and safety should be developed and established, as well as its continuous evaluation. Support and management of ambulatory orthopaedic surgery in the framework of the objectives and quality plan of any National System of Health must be consolidated.

From the perspective of the quality and efficiency there is widespread consensus on the quality, safety and efficiency of ambulatory surgery as healthcare modality. There have been indicators to know the exact value of this type of healthcare service and its quality control. The most used ones are: cancellation of procedure, Adverse events (Same-day unplanned repeated surgery, Unplanned overnight stay, Emergency consultation, Readmission to hospital, Risk-adjusted complications index), Substitution Index, Ambulatory surgery index and Satisfaction Index and postoperative pain assessment.

Disadvantages of this type of surgery, such as failure to follow perioperative instructions, inability to be served by another competent person during convalescence, the impossibility to dispose of transportation to be connected to hospital or the worry and lack of patient trust, is significantly attenuated with good patient selection.

Advantages offered by ambulatory surgery are many because of it allows more individual attention and according to the needs of the patient, altering the minimum lifestyle and allowing less disability and return to work as quickly as possible in lot of cases. Besides, it avoids all the complications of hospitalization and reduce healthcare costs.

To ensure the proper functioning and quality of this surgical modality is essential a multidisciplinary coordination and training in the techniques and requirements of day surgery in staff to be practice it communication of all professionals who are part of it. The training of practice leaders in principles of root-cause analysis, quality improvement, and process redesign is also essential so that when they receive reports of safety concerns, they are able to analyze them and enact change. Provider organizations that recognize these challenges and respond to them will be ahead of the game as the spotlight is increasingly focused on care delivered not just by hospitals but by truly accountable care organizations in all settings of care.

The complications described are rare and mild, with a low rate of unexpected admissions, without any mortal case, and good satisfaction results and overall outcome with an optimal acceptance by all those involved.

Units of ambulatory surgery require a number of structural resources and equipment, which are mainly in relation to the characteristics of the scheduled clinical activity and the degree of autonomy with regard to existing resources of each hospital centre.

Given the consolidation and advancement of ambulatory surgery in Orthopaedics, it is considered that the structural conditions of the units should be targeted to meet the requirements in good standards and recommendations, giving priority to Autonomous Units over other designs. It should be noted that the design recommendations at this respect must include functional aspects and be adapted to each specific reality. Decisions regarding the practical structure of the ambulatory units must be dependent on the organizational form and specific management of each one, and adopted, in particular, taking into account the organization and management of human resources.

Day case surgery in Orthopaedics is a very important concept which can be used to reduce the waiting time for elective operations, and help clinicians and managers to prioritize and plan patient's treatments. It needs to be incorporated in healthcare policies designs in order to minimize the hospital stay and cost, and ultimately to increase productivity.

References

[1] National Center for Health Statistics. Hospital admissions, average length of stay, and outpatient visits, according to type of ownership and size of hospital, and percent outpatient surgery: United States, selected years 1975-2000 [Table 96]. In: *Health,* United States, 2002, With Chartbook on Trends in the Health of Americans. Hyattsville, Md: NCHS; 2002.

[2] Fleisher LA, Pasternak LR, Lyles A. A novel index of elevated risk of inpatient hospital admission immediately following outpatient surgery. *Arch Surg* 2007;142:263-8.

[3] National Research and Development Centre for Welfare and Health. Care periods in 2006 and trends of care periods in the years 1997–2006. Finnish official statistics. 2007.

[4] Wu CL, Berenholtz SM, Pronovost PJ, Fleisher LA. Systematic review and analysis of postdischarge symptoms after outpatient surgery. *Anesthesiology* 2002; 96:994-1003.

[5] Punnonen H. January–December 2007 *at hospitals and hospital districts – a summary of demand, production and finance.* Helsinki: Finnish Local and Regional Authorities 34–9 2008.

[6] Mattila K, Hynynen M. Day surgery in Finland: a prospective cohort study of 14 day-surgery units. *Acta Anaesthesiol Scand* 2009; 53: 455-63.

[7] Mezei G, Chung F. Return hospital visits and hospital readmissions after ambulatory surgery. *Ann Surg* 1999; 230:721-727.

[8] Twersky R, Fishman D, Homel P. What happens after discharge? return hospital visits after ambulatory surgery. *Anesth Analg* 1997;84:319-324.

[9] Johnson CD, Jarrett PE. Admission to hospital after day case surgery. *Ann R Coll Surg Engl* 1990;72:225-228.

[10] NHS Modernisation Agency. *10 high impact changes forservice improvement and delivery: a guide for NHS leaders.* London: NHS Modernisation Agency 15–84 2004.

[11] Martin Ferrero MA, Faour Martin O. Ambulatory surgery in orthopedics: experience of over 10,000 patients. J orthopaedic science 2014; 19:332-8.

[12] American Society of Anesthesiologists Task Force on Preoperative Fasting. Practice guidelines for preoperative fasting and the use of pharmacologic agents to reduce the risk of pulmonary aspiration:

application to healthy patients undergoing elective procedures. *Anesthesiology* 1999; 90: 896–905.
[13] Korttila K. Anaesthesia for ambulatory surgery: firm definitions of "home readiness" needed. Ann Med 1991;23:635-6.
[14] Herrera FJ, Wong J, Chung MB. A Systematic Review of Postoperative Recovery Outcomes Measurements After Ambulatory Surgery. *Anesth Analg* 2007: 105: 1: 63-69.
[15] Smith I. Day surgery for all: updated selection criteria. *Current Anaesth & Critical* Care 2007; 18: 181–7.
[16] Aldwinckle RJ,Montgomery JE. Unplanned admission rates and postdischarge complications in patients over the age of 70 following day case surgery. *Anaesthesia* 2004; 59: 57–9.
[17] Ansell GL, Montgomery JE. Outcome of ASA III patientsundergoing day case surgery. *Br J Anaesth* 2004; 92: 71–4.
[18] Fortier J, Chung F, Su J. Unanticipated admission after ambulatory surgery – a prospective study. *Can J Anaesth* 1998; 45: 612–9.
[19] Coley KC, Williams BA, DaPos SV, Chen C, Smith RB.Retrospective evaluation of unanticipated admissions and readmissions after same day surgery and associated costs. *J Clin Anesth* 2002; 14: 349–53.
[20] Lindh A, Andersson AS, Westman L. Is transient lumbar pain after spinal anaesthesia with lidocaine influenced by early mobilisation? *Acta Anaesthesiol Scand* 2001: 45: 290–3.
[21] Colomer J, Ondategui S, Esteban E. Substitution indexes in ambulatory surgery: measure, count and compare. *Gac Sanit* 2001; 15:523-6.

In: Advances in Surgical Procedures
Editor: Miriam Figueroa
ISBN: 978-1-63482-461-3

Chapter 4

Free Flap Breast Reconstruction: New Updates and Refinements on a Well Established Technique

Cedric L. Hunter, MD, and Gordon K. Lee, MD, FACS*
Division of Plastic Surgery, Stanford University Medical Center, Palo Alto, California, US

Abstract

The abdominal flap is the most common method of autologous breast reconstruction worldwide. Advocates argue the predictability and ability to create a more natural breast mound exceed that of implant based reconstruction. The transverse rectus abdominis (TRAM) flap has evolved from a pedicle flap to a free myocutaneous flap, and now to a deep inferior epigastric perforator (DIEP) flap as microsurgery technique and skill has improved. Multiple recipient vessels have been used historically including the thoracodorsal, lateral thoracic, thoracoacromial, transverse cervical, and internal mammary vessels. The internal mammary artery (IMA) and vein (IMV) are common recipient vessels in today's practice as the dissection can be done quickly and their medial position allows for medial placement of the reconstructed breast mound.

* Corresponding author: Gordon Lee, MD, FACS. Stanford Plastic and Reconstructive Surgery, 770 Welch Rd, #400, Palo Alto, CA 94304-5715, Tel: 650-723-5824, fax: 650-725-6605, e-mail: glee@stanford.edu.

During the oncologic portion of the case the axillary lymph nodes are often sampled with either sentinel lymph node biopsy or variations of axillary lymph node dissections. While the axilla is a major nodal basin for breast tissue drainage some studies report as much as 20% drainage to the internal mammary lymph node basin. The dissection of the internal mammary vessels also affords an opportunity to sample internal mammary lymph nodes that may significantly alter cancer staging and treatment. Traditionally the anastomosis from the free flap to the IMA and IMV is performed in an antegrade manner with a single artery and vein. However, when additional inflow or outflow is needed an additional anastomosis can be performed in the same zone with retrograde anastomosis to the IMA and IMV with success. While the free TRAM is currently the gold standard in autologous breast reconstruction, pre-existing abdominal scars are often a deterrent to the reconstructive surgeon given concern for potential ischemic complications. Techniques involving flap design modification and supercharging or turbocharging the flaps with additional anastomoses from contralateral deep inferior epigastric vessels or superficial inferior epigastric vessels provides the reconstructive surgeon with tools for successfully managing potential problems associated with abdominal scars.

Often clinical analysis of bleeding flap edges is sufficient for assessing flap viability intraoperatively; however, new imaging modalities involving intraoperative laser-assisted indocyanine green (ICG) angiography are also being used as an adjunct to assess tissue perfusion. Other vascular imaging studies such as computed tomography angiography (CTA) are increasingly being used preoperatively to assist with perforator identification and free flap planning. The techniques discussed within this chapter highlight recent advances in perforator based microsurgery, the reconstructive surgeon's potential contribution to breast cancer staging, strategies for managing abdominal scars in abdominal based free tissue breast reconstruction, and the use of vascular imaging for the reconstructive surgeon. These techniques and tips help the reconstructive surgeon to provide excellent and predictable results while limiting complications.

Introduction

Since the birth of breast reconstruction, the reconstructive plastic surgeon has focused on developing a reliable procedure and improving aesthetic results while limiting complications and donor site morbidity. In 1982, Hartrampf brought the transverse rectus abdominis musculocutaneous (TRAM) flap to the forefront of autologous tissue breast reconstruction following mastectomy.

This technique allowed the reconstructive surgeon to utilize a transverse island of abdominal skin, subcutaneous tissue, and its underlying musculature based upon the superior epigastric vessels to recreate a natural breast mound without the need for an implant [1].

While this was an improvement to previous techniques and allowed a single stage reconstruction, there was abdominal wall morbidity due to the sacrifice of the rectus abdominis muscle. The continued evolution of technology and skill provided substantial advances that have pushed the field of breast reconstruction towards the increased utilization of free flap techniques capable of sparing abdominal muscles. The realization that the dominant blood supply to the rectus abdominis musculature and overlying abdominal wall was through the deep inferior epigastric artery and the added benefit of preserving the medial and inferior inframammary fold by avoiding tunneling of the pedicled flap also encouraged use of the free TRAM flap [2].

Current microsurgery training involves both live in operating room training in an apprenticeship model and self-directed education through interactive alternative modalities such as practice models and web-based curricula. While microsurgery training is incredibly diverse the development of reliable tools for assessing microsurgeon development is key.

One such scale for evaluating microsurgeons in training is the Stanford Microsurgery and Resident Training (SMaRT) scale, which has been validated previously [3-6]. As microsurgery techniques and training improve, the field continues to strive for improving aesthetic results and limiting donor site morbidity, which has led to the transition from the primary utilization of the free TRAM flap to utilization of the free muscle-sparing TRAM flap, the deep inferior epigastric artery perforator (DIEP) flap, and the superficial inferior epigastric artery (SIEA) flap (Figure 1 and Figure 2).

Each of these flaps utilize the same lower abdominal skin and fat as a donor site but with varying degrees of abdominal wall donor site morbidity based upon the extent of muscle that is used. Despite the varying degree of abdominal wall violation these abdominal flaps are tolerated well by the patient and in some cases have been shown to have a lower incidence of complications when compared to implant based breast reconstructions [7].

In today's practice, for autologous breast reconstruction lower abdominal tissue remains a preferred option by most reconstructive surgeons and perforator flap transfer is quickly becoming the gold standard [8]. In addition alternative non-abdominal tissue flaps including the superior gluteal artery perforator (SGAP) flap, the latissimus dorsi flap, and the transverse gracilis myocutaneous (TUG) flap all help to provide the reconstructive surgeon with a large toolbox of options for creating an aesthetic breast with autologous tissue when lower abdominal tissue is unavailable or not preferred by the patient.

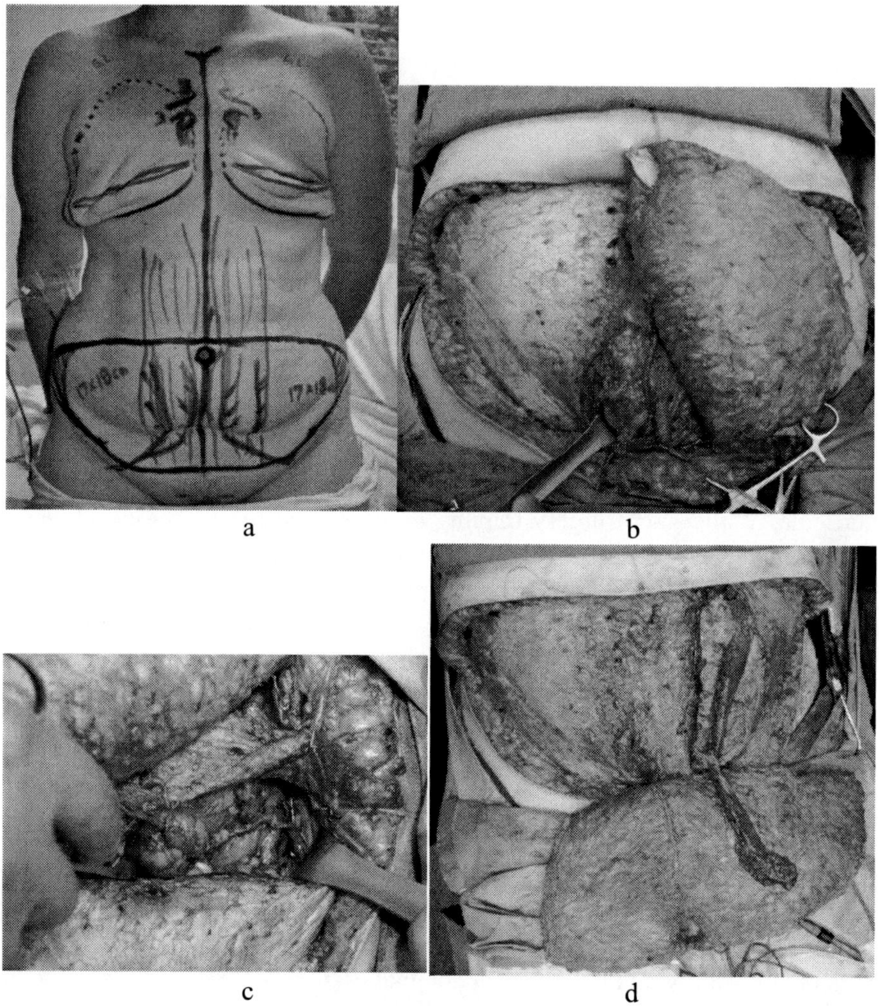

Figure 1. Free deep inferior epigastric artery flap. A) Markings used for a bilateral DIEP flap. B) After rectus sheath is opened the perforators are identified, preserved, and dissected free from the surrounding muscle back to the deep inferior epigastric artery. C) The pedicle is dissected distally. D) After flap elevation with a DIEP technique on the patient's right side and a muscle-sparing TRAM technique on the patients left side.

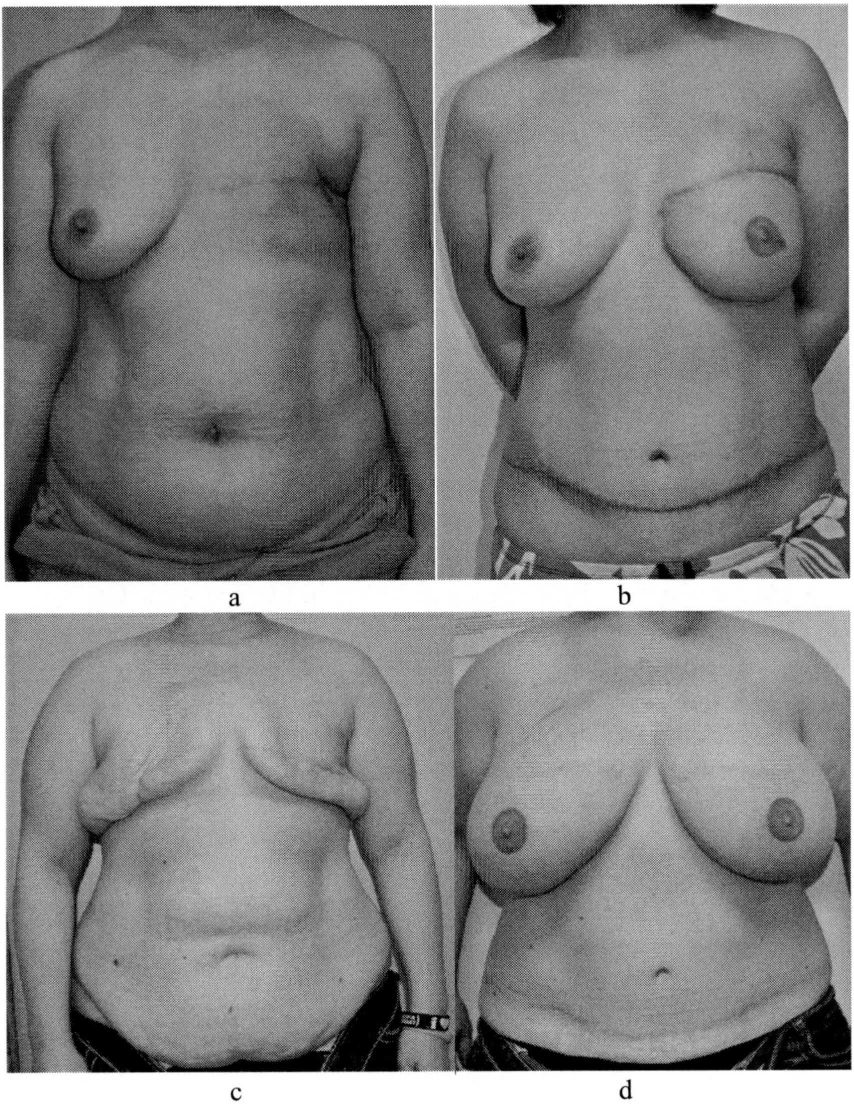

Figure 2. The final results. A) Preoperative photograph of patient with left mastectomy. B) Postoperative photograph following a left free DIEP flap and subsequent NAC reconstruction with tattooing for color. C) Preoperative photograph of patient with bilateral mastectomy defect. D) Postoperative photograph following bilateral free DIEP flap with subsequent NAC reconstruction and tattooing for color. Note significant natural ptosis consistent with patient body habitus.

Recipient Vessels

Historically, a variety of blood vessels have been used as potential recipient vessels for microvascular anastomosis in free flap breast reconstruction. Recipient arteries have included internal mammary, thoracodorsal, thoracoacromial, posterior humeral circumflex, circumflex scapular, and the axillary artery. Recipient veins have included internal mammary, thoracodorsal, cephalic vein of the arm, axillary vein branches, thoracoacromial vein, scapular circumflex, and the axillary vein [9]. While the use of the axillary, scapular circumflex, and thoracoacromial vessels are infrequent; they can serve as lifeboats in the event of damage and unavailability of the primary planned vessels. The thoracoacromial vessels supply the pectoralis major muscle and can be found below the clavicle in the midclavicular region on the undersurface of the pectoralis major muscle. The circumflex scapular vessels are found where they join the thoracodorsal vessels to form the subscapular system. Tracing the subscapular system in a retrograde fashion into the axilla identifies the axillary vessels. Care must be taken to avoid traction injury to the brachial plexus during this dissection. Currently, the two most common recipient vessel sites for free tissue breast reconstruction are the thoracodorsal and internal mammary vessels.

In the case of immediate breast reconstruction following modified radical mastectomy in which axillary lymph node sampling is performed, the thoracodorsal vessels are either fully or partially exposed by the oncologic resection requiring minimal preparation by the reconstructive surgeon. Ideally, the reconstructed breast mound position should be medial enough to create medial fullness and cleavage for improved aesthetics. This is often difficult to achieve with anastomosis to the thoracodorsal vessels given their lateral location in the axilla. For improved results the thoracodorsal vessels must be dissected free not only from the surrounding tissue, but also freed from the branches to the serratus muscle to the level of the scapular circumflex vessels for sufficient length. In addition, for successful mound placement with use of the thoracodorsal vessels a long donor pedicle is needed.

Today, many surgeons prefer to use the internal mammary vessels as recipient vessels for breast reconstruction. This mirrors a change in the increased use of sentinel lymph node biopsy over axillary lymph node dissection for clinically uninvolved axillary lymph nodes. There are notable benefits to using the internal mammary vessels as primary recipients. In delayed reconstruction fresh tissue planes with lack of perivascular scarring from previous operations decreases the risk of damaging the recipient vessels during exposure. In delayed or immediate reconstruction the more medial position of the flap improves aesthetics and provides better positioning for vessel anastomosis [10, 11]. In cases of delayed axillary dissection after sentinel lymph node biopsy an internal mammary anastomosis circumvents possible damage to the pedicle, which would be at significant risk had the thoracodorsal vessels been used. Furthermore internal mammary vessel use as recipient vessels broadens the reconstructive surgeons flap options, as a shorter pedicle length can be accommodated and still allow medial placement of the flap while limiting lateral fullness [12].

The senior author prefers to use the internal mammary vessels as first-line recipient vessels for breast reconstruction when available (Figure 3). The internal mammary vessels are approached by elevating a flap of pectoralis major muscle overlying the third rib exposing the underlying rib and intercostal muscles. The perichondrium of the third rib is then incised along the anterior surface of the costal cartilage from the sternal junction to the costochondral junction. Blunt and sharp dissection is used to separate the perichondrium from the underlying cartilage on the anterior and posterior surface. The cartilage is then removed with a rongeur. The deep perichondrium is then incised and reflected from lateral to medial. Bipolar electrocautery and hemoclips are used to control small branches from the internal mammary vessels. Care must be taken to avoid injury to the underlying pleura and lung during the dissection. Once the internal mammary vessels are identified the exposure is increased by dividing the intercostal musculature from the second to the fourth rib. The internal mammary vein tends to be larger on the right side compared to the left. It is important to select the appropriate costal cartilage for removal as the internal mammary veins decrease in size and bifurcate at or below the fourth interspace making venous anastomosis more difficult below this level [10]. After adequate exposure the vessels are generally divided at the level of the fourth rib for sufficient length during microscopic anastomosis (Figure 4). While the use of the internal mammary vessels in free flap breast reconstruction is becoming more widespread, it is not without its drawbacks. One particular drawback is that after the internal mammary vessels are used for breast reconstruction, they are no longer available for use as an arterial conduit in coronary revascularization. Studies have noted that the incidence of cardiovascular disease in women with breast cancer who have undergone free flap breast reconstruction is quite low as women with pre-existing coronary artery disease or significant comorbidities are likely to undergo a more simple operation such as implant based reconstruction.

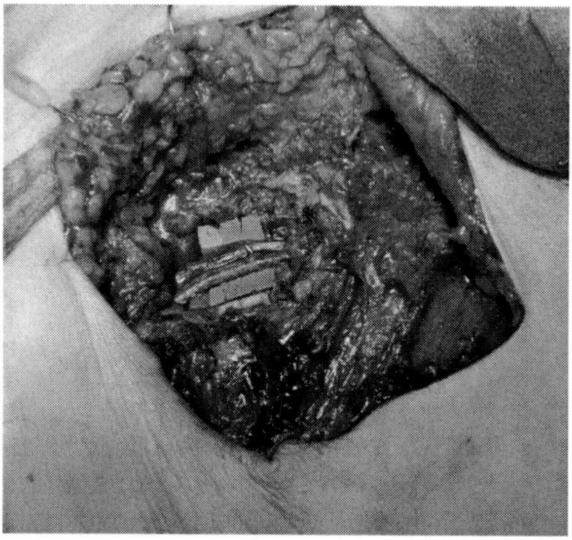

Figure 3. Exposed internal mammary artery and vein.

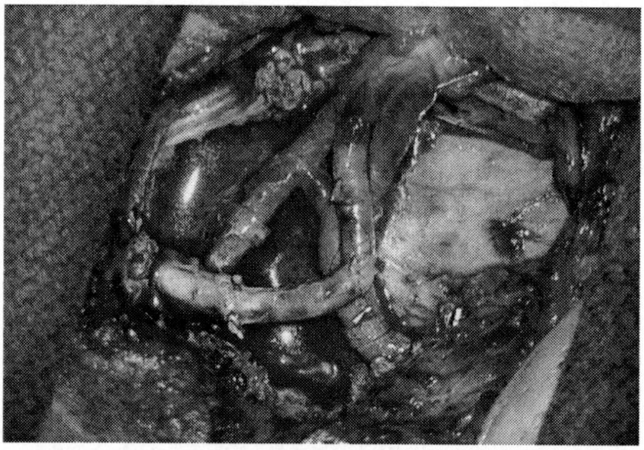

Figure 4. Free flap anastomosis to internal mammary artery and vein.

Additionally the increasing use of percutaneous angioplasty procedures decreases the need for mammary bridge in coronary revascularization. Overall, the use of internal mammary vessel use in breast reconstruction surgery is quite safe; however, this potential drawback should be discussed with the patient [13].

Vascular Optimization

Venous Outflow

After vessel anastomosis and flap inset, one major complication that can be seen with free flap breast reconstruction is venous congestion. DIEP flap venous congestion is multifactorial and is influenced by patient factors (i.e., smoking history, obesity, etc.), technical expertise, and anatomy of the venous system. The reconstructive surgeon must be cognizant and capable of managing potential venous outflow complications that could comprise the reconstructed breast. In the past there were reports of managing venous congestion with cephalic vein harvest and transfer to augment venous drainage and reduce necrosis as either primary venous drainage or additional venous drainage [14]. Significant advances in the understanding of the venous drainage system of the lower abdominal tissues as well as the internal mammary vascular system has allowed for improved methods of augmenting and managing venous drainage after flap transfer.

Anatomic studies of abdominal based tissue flaps have noted that the superficial inferior epigastric vein (SIEV) or deep inferior epigastric vein (DIEV) alone may not be fully capable of supporting drainage of the entire flap leading to venous congestion if not appropriately addressed. If congestion is appreciated intra-operatively this is addressed with 1) separate anastomoses of the DIEV and the SIEV, or 2) if truly one system is dominant (superficial vs. deep) then single anastomosis of the dominant system with or without vein graft is justified. The senior author has reported harvesting the DIEV as a vein graft in cases of SIEV dominance when additional vein length is needed [15]. When needed there are several sources of additional drainage include the external jugular vein, external facial vein, thoracodorsal vein, etc. [14, 16, 17]. When performing primary anastomosis to the internal mammary vessels, one often appreciates that the internal mammary vein has already branched at the level of the anastomosis. In this case, the venous flow can be augmented by utilizing this paired system and performing additional venous anastomosis with SIEV or contralateral DIEV to this second internal mammary vein. In the absence of a branched or paired internal mammary vein another attractive option is to join the superficial and deep drainage systems by performing and additional anastomosis between the DIEV and the SIEV for venous augmentation. Yet another option, and that preferred by the senior author, in the absence of paired internal mammary veins is to perform independent antegrade and retrograde anastomosis to the internal mammary vein after division. We have experienced successful results with utilization of the distal internal mammary vein stump at our institution and there are a few series that have also reported positive results with this technique [18, 19]. Previous studies have noted or assumed that the lack of valves in the internal mammary veins contribute to the success of internal mammary vein use as a conduit in either an antegrade or retrograde fashion [20, 21]. On the contrary, Mackey et al. performed an anatomic study of the internal mammary veins and noted that 43% of cadavers had valves in at least one vein or major branch. They suggested that given the reported success it was likely that bulk of retrograde flow in the IMV occurs through collaterals and communicating side branches, or valve incompetence allowing regurgitant flow [22]. Options for antegrade and retrograde anastomosis include: 1) In the case of DIEP vena comitans, the larger can be anastomosed to the proximal limb in an antegrade fashion and the smaller can be anastomosed to the distal limb in an retrograde fashion; 2) the deep inferior epigastric vein can be anastomosed to the proximal limb and the SIEV can be anastomosed to the distal limb in a retrograde fashion; and 3) for bipedicled DIEP flaps the internal mammary vein can again be used in an antegrade and retrograde fashion. By utilizing the internal mammary vein for retrograde flow, distal vein grafts and morbidity associated with additional dissection can be avoided. The retrograde use of the internal mammary vein provides another avenue for flap salvage, venous supercharging, and double pedicle reconstruction when appropriate. These all highlight the importance of preserving the SIEV on both sides and obtaining maximal length during the initial dissection. When no additional outflow can be established in venous congestion, leech therapy is considered for venous decompression to avoid venous stasis and thrombosis.

Arterial Inflow

While retrograde use of the internal mammary vein provides an additional option for venous drainage, retrograde anastomosis to the internal mammary artery provides the reconstructive surgeon with a means for augmenting vascular inflow to the flap. While the first choice for autogenous tissue breast reconstruction is the single pedicle flap, there are circumstances where similar to the need for increased venous drainage the reconstructive surgeon will be faced with a need for increased arterial in-flow. The increase in arterial inflow often comes in the form of a double pedicle flap. In 1990, Hartrampf et al. described the benefit of the double-pedicle TRAM: 1) in the presence of a midline scar when reconstruction requires greater tissue than that contained in the hemi-abdomen, 2) when the volume of the tissue needed for reconstruction was large and exceeded that which could reliably be carried on a single pedicle, and 3) those at high risk for partial flap necrosis [23]. The use of bilateral rectus muscles for bi-pedicled flaps resulted in significant abdominal wall morbidity [24]. Other techniques involving "supercharging" or "turbocharging" were developed to improve blood flow in the uni-pedicled flap. In the "supercharged" flap the deep inferior epigastric vessels or the superficial inferior epigastric vessels were anastomosed to independent and unrelated source vessels in the axilla such as the thoracodorsal vessels [25, 26]. Whereas, in the "turbocharged" flap the vascular augmentation was provided by a source vessel already intrinsic to the flap such as anastomosis of the deep inferior epigastric vessels to each other creating a loop [27]. As the use of free flaps increased techniques such as the bipedicled free TRAM flap with anastomosis to the thoracodorsal and serratus collateral vessels increased in popularity [28]. As changes in reconstructive surgery technique often mirrors change in technique of the extirpative surgeon, decreased axillary dissection resulted in an increase of internal mammary artery use for recipient vessels and a movement away from combining internal mammary vessels and axillary vessels for bipedicled free flaps to the use of internal mammary vessels alone with two sets of microvascular anastomosis to the proximal and distal ends of the transected internal mammary vessels [29, 30]. When vascular augmentation is needed for DIEP flap breast reconstruction the senior author prefers to utilize the proximal and distal cut ends of the internal mammary vessels for anastomoses to the deep inferior epigastric vessels or superficial inferior epigastric vessels in an end-to-end fashion. The retrograde flow through the distal cut end has been observed to provide sufficient flow for needed augmentation.

Management of Abdominal Scars

The presence of pre-existing abdominal scars presents a challenge to the reconstructive surgeon as the scars can place the free flap or remaining abdominal wall tissues at risk for necrosis. The presence of an abdominal scar requires the reconstructive surgeon to recognize the potential challenge to tissue perfusion and make necessary modifications to flap design and/or harvest technique to mitigate complications. There are extreme cases where multiple abdominal scars may be a contraindication to surgery; however, abdominal scars in and of themselves are not absolute contraindications to abdominal tissue based autologous breast reconstruction. As mentioned, Hartrampf noted early on that patients with large tissue requirements and a midline abdominal scar benefited from double pedicle TRAM flaps [23]. This technique resulted in considerable abdominal wall weakness after the harvest of bilateral rectus abdominis muscles [31]. Other techniques for vascular augmentation were developed to prevent flap necrosis. Berrino originally described the "Parasite TRAM Flap" which involved harvesting a unilateral superiorly based pedicled TRAM flap and utilizing retrograde flow from the ipsilateral deep inferior epigastric vessels to supply the contralateral deep inferior epigastric vessels [32]. As free flap breast reconstruction became more prevalent others have compensated for the loss of volume by stacking free hemi-DIEP flaps with varying recipient vessels for antegrade and retrograde flow in the presence of a midline abdominal scar [33, 34]. There have been numerous modifications for in-flap vascular augmentation across midline scars that have included anastomosing a premuscular branch off the main deep inferior epigastric artery pedicle across the midline to the proximal end of the contralateral deep inferior epigastric vessels, or creating an anastomosis between the stump of the superior epigastric vessels to contralateral paraumbilical perforators [35-37].

The senior author prefers to use the DIEP flap as a first choice to create an aesthetic breast despite the presence of abdominal scars. With necessary adjustments in flap design and harvest the DIEP flap is safely done in patients with pre-existing abdominal scars. We routinely identify the superficial inferior epigastric vessels intraoperatively and dissect them for a minimum of 4-5 cm through the subcutaneous tissue for added length. These vessels are then preserved for possible later use. A recent anatomic study notes a 94% incidence of the SIEA on CTA; however, only 24% had a diameter > 1.5 mm. The SIEV was present in all cases [38]. The identification and preservation of these vessels when possible affords the reconstructive surgeon added flexibility for managing pre-existing abdominal wall scars. Each case is to be considered based on a number of factors including, the location of the abdominal scar, whether the reconstruction is unilateral or bilateral, and the volume of tissue needed for a symmetric reconstruction.

In the case of a midline infra-umbilical scar, a patient needing a unilateral reconstruction in the presence of a large and pendulous native breast, the reconstruction will require a large amount of tissue often crossing the midline and preventing the use of a hemi-DIEP flap. In this case a bipedicled DIEP flap is harvested to provide perfusion on both sides of the scar.

Other viable options include a DIEP pedicle on one side and an SIEA pedicle on the other side, or a bipedicled SIEA flap if a smaller volume is required (Figure 5). For bilateral reconstructions or small volume unilateral reconstructions the midline scar marks the medial edge of the flap. In cases of a midline supra-umbilical scar, there is no change in flap design; however, the scar can tether the skin to the fascia making donor site closure difficult. Complete undermining of the skin and subcutaneous tissue flaps to the xiphoid past the scar should eliminate this problem.

The paramedian scar is encountered less frequently, yet can be a cause of significant morbidity if not addressed appropriately. For bilateral and unilateral cases one must ensure that there are perforators on each side of the scar. In unilateral breast reconstruction we preferentially harvest a bipedicled DIEP flap and proceed if the scar is medial to the lateral perforators. In bilateral cases or when the scar is located lateral to the deep inferior epigastric perforators we utilize the superficial inferior epigastric vessels to supercharge or turbocharge the flap for blood supply across the scar [39]. In these cases we prefer to perform two independent anastomoses to the proximal and distal cut ends of the internal mammary artery and vein limiting the need for further dissection into the axilla to access the thoracodorsal vessels [34] (Figure 6).

With a pre-existing low transverse or pfannenstiel incision scar the flap is positioned more inferiorly so that the scar becomes the inferior border of the flap. Flap dissection and vessel selection may then usually proceed as planned. In theory the perforators and deep inferior epigastric vessels are preserved as Pfannenstiel's original description describes a transverse skin incision with vertical splitting of the rectus muscles through the linea alba to access the pelvis [40, 41]. Despite this description it is prudent to fully evaluate for intact source vessels prior to completing flap harvest, as it is not uncommon to encounter transected muscle and source vessels or an undermined flap with damage to abdominal wall perforators jeopardizing the ability to safely harvest an abdominal flap. If there is any question of perforator viability the flap should be harvested as either an MS-TRAM or free TRAM flap.

The subcostal scar, often used for open cholecystectomy, if low enough can be incorporated as a superior edge of the flap. When the scar is too high to incorporate into the incision modifications are made to both flap design and harvest. While the deep inferior epigastric vessels are remote from the scar, ... a key role in providing perfusion to the abdominal tissue below the ... rectus muscle and superior epigastric arteries have been ... est of the deep inferior epigastric artery places the remaining ... at risk for ischemic complications.

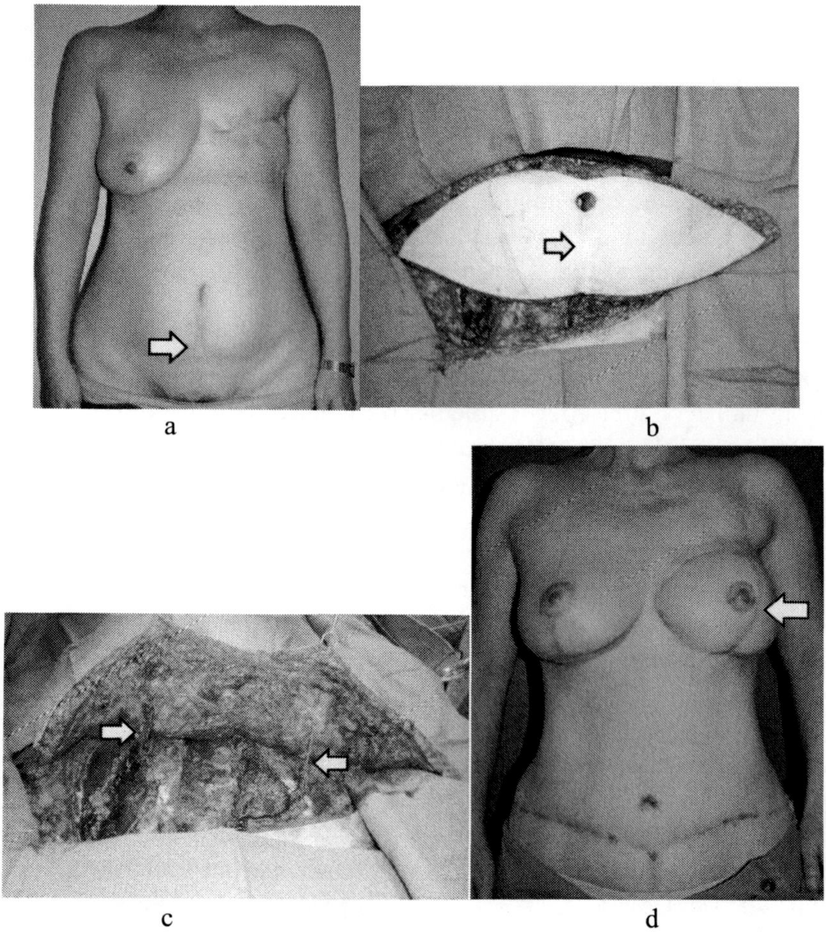

Figure 5. Midline infraumbilical scar. A) Preoperative photograph of a patient with midline infraumbilical scar and left mastectomy defect. B) Intraoperative photograph of harvested abdominal tissue flap. C) Intraoperative photograph of bipedicled DIEP flap, pedicles marked with arrows. D) Postoperative photograph of patient with a bipedicled DIEP flap for left breast reconstruction and right breast mastopexy for symmetry.

In this case the designed peaks of the abdominal flap are lower than normal and the flap is smaller to preserve a broad base of tissue beneath the scar to perfuse the remaining skin flap. Undermining of the skin and subcutaneous flap near the scar is limited to only that what is needed for tension free closure in an effort to preserve nearby perforators to the sk (Figure 7).

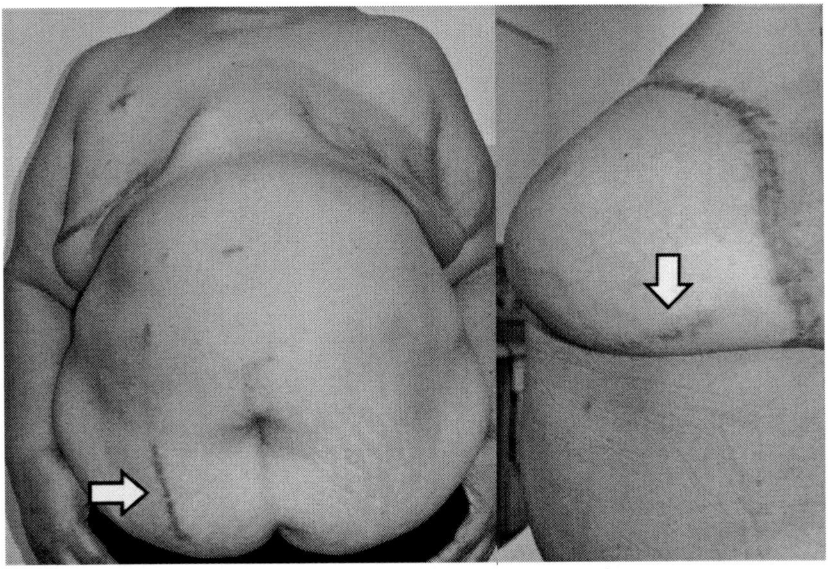

a b

Figure 6. Paramedian scar. A) Preoperative photograph of a patient with a right paramedian scar and bilateral mastectomy defects. B) Postoperative photograph of patient with bilateral DIEP flap breast reconstruction. The left breast is reconstructed with a bipedicled DIEP and SIEA flap to preserve as much volume as possible.

Right lower quadrant or McBurney's incisions for open appendectomy result in abdominal scars that could compromise the lateral edges of the DIEP flap. In these cases if the orientation and location of the scar is amenable, it is best served to shift the flap so that the scar marks the inferolateral edge of the flap. When this is not possible and the scar has to be included to increase flap volume the SIEA and SIEV are available to supercharge or turbocharge the flap and perfuse the area across the scar (Figure 8).

If the SIEA and SIEV are unavailable and there are ischemic concerns beyond the scar excision of the ischemic portion of the flap is recommended. Although there has been no demonstrated increase of flap or donor site complications for DIEP flaps in the presence of abdominal scars from laparoscopic port placement, port scars in the vicinity of the vascular pedicle and perforators can increase the technical difficulty of the dissection [42].

The key when performing autologous breast reconstruction with abdominal tissue in the presence of pre-existing abdominal scars is providing independent perfusion on both sides of the scar.

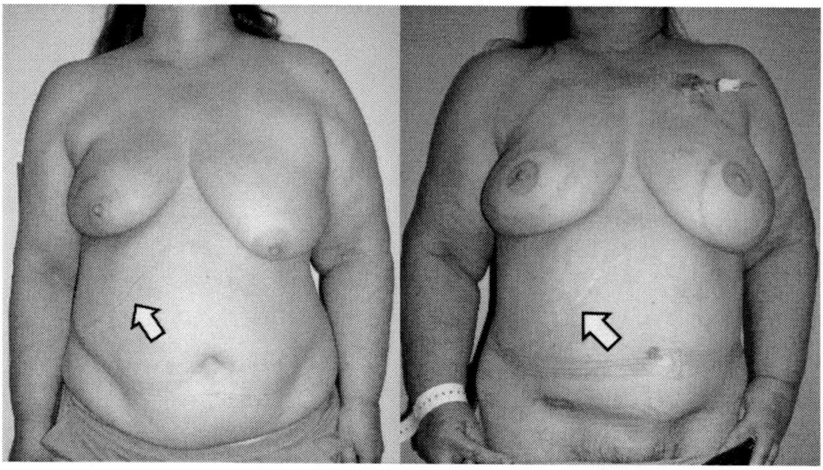

a b

Figure 7. Subcostal scar. A) Preoperative photograph of a patient with a right subcostal scar and right breast cancer. B) Postoperative photograph after patient has undergone bilateral mastectomy and bilateral DIEP flap breast reconstruction with subsequent NAC reconstruction and tattooing for color.

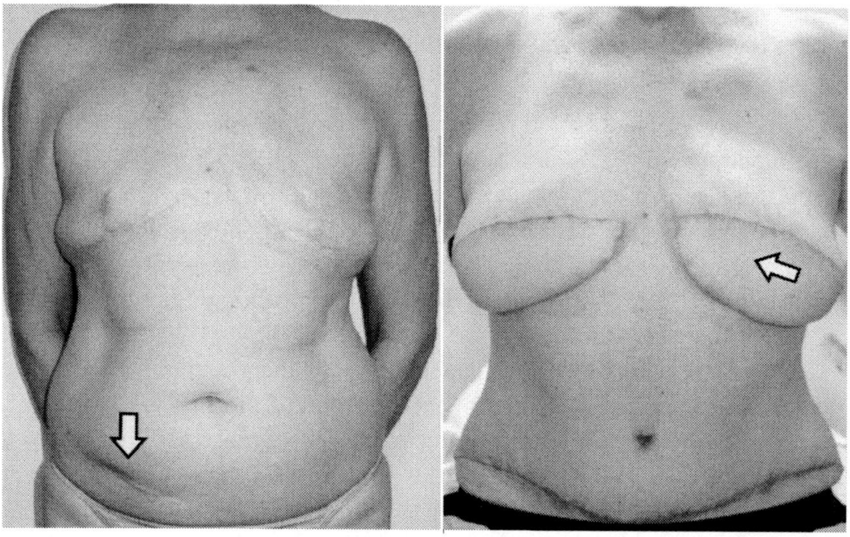

a b

Figure 8. Right lower quadrant scar. A) Preoperative photograph of a patient with a right lower quadrant scar from a McBurney's incision and bilateral mastectomy defects. B) Postoperative photograph after bilateral DIEP flap breast reconstruction. She has yet to undergo NAC reconstruction.

Tissue perfusion should be assessed intraoperatively for final decision-making and any evidence of venous or arterial insufficiency should prompt vascular supplementation.

Imaging

There has been a growing popularity for the use of preoperative and intraoperative imaging amongst breast reconstructive surgeons. The most critical aspect of designing and harvesting the DIEP flap is determining the amount of viable tissue that can safely be harvested on a particular perforator. Doppler sonography with or without color duplex imaging has been used to localize cutaneous perforators with high sensitivity allowing preoperative identification. Qualitative assessments based on the harshness of the sound provided a subjective comparison for perforator dominance within a certain skin territory [43, 44]. However, Doppler sonography has its drawbacks including detecting vessels that may be too small to support a given skin flap, inability to identify location of perforator take off, and operator dependence [45]. Due to increased detail and reproducibility, preoperative imaging in the form of computed tomography angiography (CTA) has largely supplanted previously used color duplex sonography in assisting with the planning and selection of perforators for flap harvest. Multidetector-row computed tomography (MDCT) is a recent innovation that allows rapid simultaneous acquisition of multiple thin collimated slices with high spatial resolution and low artifact. The time of acquisition is 10-12 seconds and the total procedure time takes about 10 minutes to perform. The data is then used to reconstruct 1 mm slices and reformatted images in multiple planes (coronal, axial, sagittal, and oblique) as well as a three-dimensional volume reconstruction [46]. Reports suggest that with CTA perforator mapping operative times and postoperative complications associated with partial necrosis of the flap are decreased [47, 48]. In addition to its utility in evaluating free flap donor site anatomy, CTA can also be used to evaluate recipient site anatomy and detect vascular anomalies that can alter the surgical plan, particularly in the cases of traumatic injury reconstructive procedures [49]. While there is acknowledgement that CTA can indeed accurately identify perforators and provide a roadmap for the surgeon there are drawbacks with regard to radiation exposure, need for intravenous contrast media, and increased cost. In a recent study by Mathes et al., they noted that 44% of abdominal perforator flaps involved intraoperative changes due to features not seen on preoperative

CT imaging that resulted in the use of additional perforators that were not a part of the initial preoperative plan or the abandonment of initially planned perforators. They noted that while CTA does provide an excellent roadmap for surgical planning and can facilitate flap dissection, it is not a panacea for free flap breast reconstruction. The surgeon must consider not only the anatomical aspects, but also the functional aspects such as location, intramuscular course, and intervening muscle between perforators [50].

More recently, magnetic resonance angiography (MRA) has shown promise in perforator imaging. High field 3-Tesla MRA is capable of producing detailed, multiplanar images, and three-dimensional reconstruction without the associated radiation exposure seen in CT imaging.

Some have utilized blood-pool contrast agents such as gadofosveset trisodium for contrast-enhanced MRA. Reportedly, gadofosveset trisodium is retained in the intravascular space resulting in higher spatial resolution, in contrast to the conventional gadolinium-based contrast [51]. This technology is in its early stages and still requires further investigation. In general, preoperative imaging when used should not replace or supersede clinical judgment, but can be used as an adjunct for the reconstructive surgeon in preoperative planning. At this time the necessity of and clinical utility of preoperative imaging remains a topic of debate. Currently, we do not routinely obtain preoperative imaging studies.

With regard to intraoperative imaging, there are new imaging modalities such as intraoperative laser-assisted indocyanine green (ICG) angiography that are being used as an adjunct to help assess tissue perfusion. Inadequate tissue perfusion is one of the known key causes to early complications in free flap surgery [52] (Figure 9). To identify areas of decreased perfusion, laser assisted ICG angiography begins with intravenous injection of ICG fluorescent dye, which binds to plasma proteins confining the dye to the intravascular compartment as it travels rapidly through the vascular system. The dye fluoresces at 806 nm. Following stimulation with laser energy the fluorescence pattern can be captured on a charge-coupled device camera or monitor for dynamic and real time images in the operating room [53, 54]. Similarly, fluorescein has been used in the past as a perfusion marker; however, capillary leakage, and prolonged clearance of 12-18 hours limited its utility as a useful intraoperative tool [55, 56]. In contrast, ICG is not as susceptible to capillary leakage and with increased clearance repetitive dye administration may occur after 9 minutes for perfusion re-evaluation [54]. The infrared laser and ICG are capable of demonstrating dermal and superficial soft tissue perfusion to a depth of approximately 3.6 mm [57].

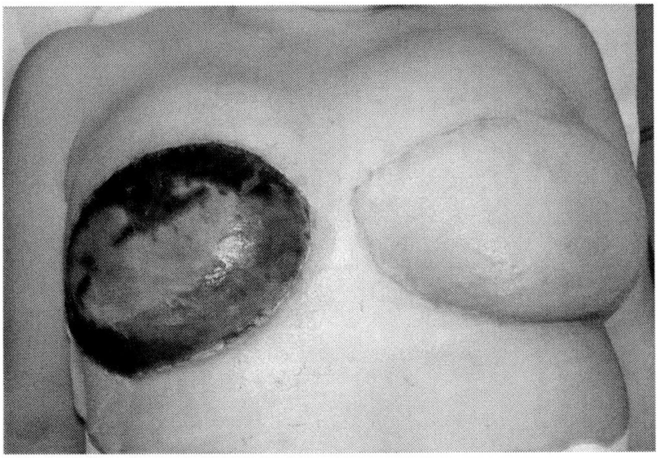

a

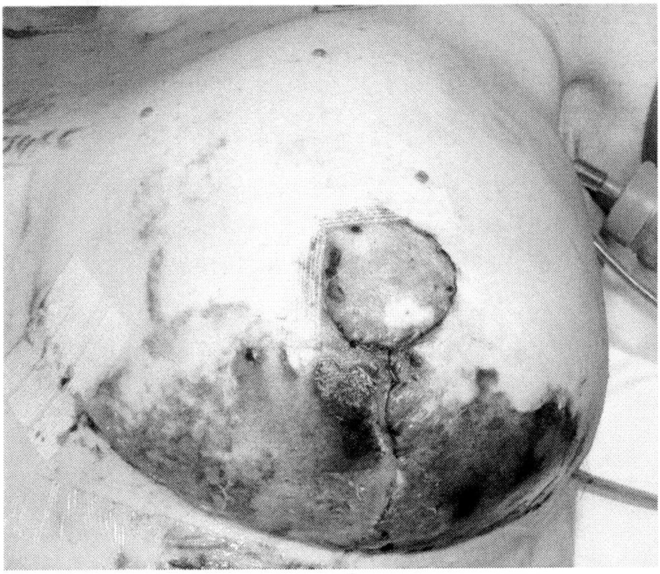

b

Figure 9. Ischemic complications. A) Flap ischemia of the right reconstructed breast that will require debridement and alternative reconstruction. B) Ischemia of lower breast skin flaps in breast reconstruction.

This technology has wide applicability to the plastic surgeon for evaluation of all components of the flap including, skin, fat, fascia, muscle, and nipples in breast reconstruction, and arterial and venous flow in microsurgery [58] (Figure 10).

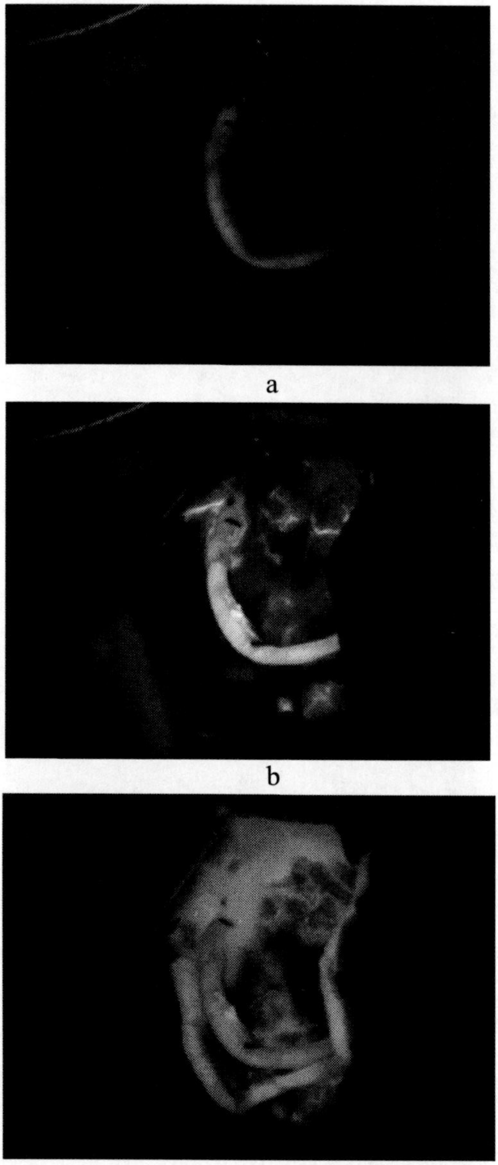

c

Figure 10. Laser-assisted indocyanine green angiography. A) An initial low intensity signal is seen in the artery. B) A stronger intensity signal is seen in the artery to the flap as the ICG continues to be distributed throughout the vascular system. C) As blood containing ICG perfuses and exits the flap a signal is now seen in the vein.

A major drawback with any form of vascular imaging is that the observed imaging only produces a single snapshot of perfusion at a given time. For ICG angiography in particular, while the surgeon may obtain real-time qualitative data with regards to flap perfusion at time point zero, ICG angiography cannot account for resolved vasospasm or the opening of "choke vessels" at a later time point. Blindly accepting that areas of decreased perfusion on ICG angiography are and will remain ischemic and later necrotic could result in resection of tissue that may have survived with more time. While this modality has been correlated with clinical outcomes and has been used for surgical decision-making, at this time there are no quantitative perfusion thresholds above which tissue survival can be anticipated. Interestingly, in the rat model, skin necrosis has been appreciated when perfusion was less than 25% of reference skin and delayed wound healing was seen in a human study with a signal of less than 60% of normal skin [56, 59]. This technology remains in its initial phases and more basic work is needed in defining the correlation between tissue perfusion and necrosis to develop predictive guidelines and strategies for clinical use. At this time while clinical judgment of the flap based on tissue color, capillary refill, flap temperature, and dermal bleeding may inaccurately assess the adequacy of tissue perfusion; it remains the most common method of flap blood supply evaluation [60].

Reconstructive surgeons are constantly looking for ways to improve free flap outcomes, as free flap loss can be catastrophic. Ideally, the surgeon could identify simple, reliable, and accurate adjunctive modalities that allow early intervention and limit postoperative complications. At this time no imaging modality has satisfied all of these criteria; however, as the use of promising innovative technologies such as intraoperative ICG angiography continue to grow and improve they could ultimately prove invaluable in decreasing complications due to ischemic causes.

Internal Mammary Lymph Nodes

Historically, the extended radical mastectomy involved axillary and internal mammary (IM) lymph node dissection with studies demonstrating a 20-30% incidence of IM nodal disease in breast cancer [61]. A randomized trial comparing radical mastectomy with extended radical mastectomy demonstrated no significant survival benefit of an extended procedure that was associated with significant morbidity. They did however note the prognostic value of the IM nodes as mortality rates of IM nodal involvement alone was similar to that of axillary nodal involvement alone, while involvement of both locations was associated with a significantly higher mortality [62]. The dissection of IM nodes has since been largely abandoned. On the other hand, axillary lymph node disease is a well-established prognostic indicator and predictor of survival in breast cancer. Reports suggest that 20-30% of node negative patients will develop recurrence within 10 years compared to approximately 70% of those with axillary nodal disease [63]. Traditionally axillary nodal status was established by axillary lymph node dissections [64]. However, development of sentinel lymph node (SLN) biopsy, where the first lymph nodes receiving lymphatic drainage from the primary tumor are selectively sampled with radioactive or blue dye, has rapidly emerged as a less morbid alternative to axillary dissection. In fact, sentinel lymph node biopsy is now regarded as the standard of care in patients without clinical or radiographic evidence of nodal disease in early-stage breast cancer [64, 65].

As Halstedian mastectomies have now fallen out of favor for modified radical and total mastectomies, and imaging technologies have improved allowing for sentinel lymph node biopsies the question of IM nodal management has again presented itself. A recent study evaluating the rate of metastasis to the IM nodal basin and the clinical implications noted a visualization of IM SLNs in 22% of patients using preoperative lymphoscintigraphy. Of those nodes that were surgically removed, they noted that 25% were positive for metastatic disease. Clinically, based on tumor-positive IM SLNs, 7% of those patients that underwent IM SLN biopsy had a change in their treatment regimen of radiation or chemotherapy [66]. Internal mammary lymph node biopsy can be done through a parasternal incision at a selected intercostal space with or without partial rib removal. Given the low numbers of patients that require changes to their systemic or radiation therapy regimen, some consider the biopsy unnecessary [67]. As mentioned above, with decreasing axillary dissections the reconstructive surgeon has transitioned from use of axillary vessels to primary use of internal mammary vessels as recipient vessels for free flap breast reconstruction. During this procedure a partial rib resection is routine and IM lymph nodes are often immediately accessible. The senior author routinely samples these lymph nodes with no time added to the case and no additional morbidity. We contend that biopsy of these nodes is important and should not be overlooked. Ideally, the biopsied nodes provide more accurate staging of breast cancer. Particularly those patients with involvement of the IM nodes with no disease in the axillary nodes and no high-risk features that would indicate the need for systemic therapy or those without metastases to the IM nodes that would lead to sparing the potential toxicity of parasternal IM node irradiation would benefit the most [68]. In this manner the reconstructive surgeon not only contributes to the breast reconstruction, but to the oncologic treatment as well as the information obtained from the IM lymph node biopsy taken in the context of other clinical factors such as axillary node status, age, tumor features, etc. will help guide further adjuvant therapies needed beyond breast reconstruction.

References

[1] Scheflan, M., Hartrampf, C. R., Black, P. W. Breast reconstruction with a transverse abdominal island flap. *Plastic and reconstructive surgery*. 1982;69(5):908-9. Epub. 1982/05/01. PubMed PMID: 7071252.

[2] Scheflan, M., Dinner, M. I. The transverse abdominal island flap: part I. Indications, contraindications, results, and complications. *Annals of plastic surgery*. 1983;10(1):24-35. Epub. 1983/01/01. PubMed PMID: 6219607.

[3] Satterwhite, T., Son, J., Carey, J., Echo, A., Spurling, T., Paro, J., et al. The Stanford Microsurgery and Resident Training (SMaRT) Scale: validation of an on-line global rating scale for technical assessment. *Annals of plastic surgery*. 2014;72 Suppl. 1:S84-8. Epub. 2014/04/03. doi: 10.1097/SAP.0000000000000139. PubMed PMID: 24691332.

[4] Satterwhite, T., Son, J., Carey, J., Zeidler, K., Bari, S., Gurtner, G., et al. Microsurgery education in residency training: validating an online curriculum. *Annals of plastic surgery*. 2012;68(4):410-4. Epub. 2012/03/ 17. doi: 10.1097/SAP.0b013e31823b6a1a. PubMed PMID: 22421490.

[5] Nykiel, M., Wong, R., Lee, G. An economical training model to teach and practice deep inferior epigastric artery perforator dissection. *Annals of plastic surgery*. 2014;72 Suppl. 1:S66-70. Epub 2014/04/18. doi: 10.1097/SAP.0000000000000176. PubMed PMID: 24740027.

[6] Son, J., Zeidler, K. R., Echo, A., Otake, L., Ahdoot, M., Lee, G. K. Teaching Core Competencies of Reconstructive Microsurgery With the Use of Standardized Patients. *Annals of plastic surgery*. 2013. Epub. 2013/03/15. doi: 10.1097/SAP.0b013e3182853f2c. PubMed PMID: 234 86137.

[7] Liu, C., Momeni, A., Zhuang, Y., Luan, J., Chung, M. T., Wright, E., et al. Outcome analysis of expander/implant versus microsurgical abdominal flap breast reconstruction: a critical study of 254 cases.

Annals of surgical oncology. 2014;21(6):2074-82. Epub. 2014/02/22. doi: 10.1245/s10434-014-3521-0. PubMed PMID: 24558063.

[8] Yu, S. C., Kleiber, G. M., Song, D. H. An algorithmic approach to total breast reconstruction with free tissue transfer. *Archives of plastic surgery*. 2013;40(3):173-80. Epub. 2013/06/05. doi: 10.5999/aps.2013.40.3.173. PubMed PMID: 23730589; PubMed Central PMCID: PMC 3665857.

[9] Shaw, W. W. Breast reconstruction by superior gluteal microvascular free flaps without silicone implants. *Plastic and reconstructive surgery*. 1983;72(4):490-501. Epub. 1983/10/01. PubMed PMID: 6611775.

[10] Clark, C. P., 3rd, Rohrich, R. J., Copit, S., Pittman, C. E., Robinson, J. An anatomic study of the internal mammary veins: clinical implications for free-tissue-transfer breast reconstruction. *Plastic and reconstructive surgery*. 1997;99(2):400-4. Epub. 1997/02/01. PubMed PMID: 9030147.

[11] Feller, A. M., Galla, T. J. The deep inferior epigastric artery perforator flap. *Clinics in plastic surgery*. 1998;25(2):197-206. Epub. 1998/06/17. PubMed PMID: 9627777.

[12] Dupin, C. L., Allen, R. J., Glass, C. A., Bunch, R. The internal mammary artery and vein as a recipient site for free-flap breast reconstruction: a report of 110 consecutive cases. *Plastic and reconstructive surgery*. 1996;98(4):685-9; discussion 90-2. Epub. 1996/09/01. PubMed PMID: 8773691.

[13] Nahabedian, M. Y. The internal mammary artery and vein as recipient vessels for microvascular breast reconstruction: are we burning a future bridge? *Annals of plastic surgery*. 2004;53(4):311-6. Epub. 2004/09/24. PubMed PMID: 15385762.

[14] Barnett, G. R., Carlisle, I. R., Gianoutsos, M. P. The cephalic vein: an aid in free TRAM flap breast reconstruction. Report of 12 cases. *Plastic and reconstructive surgery*. 1996;97(1):71-6; discussion 7-8. Epub. 1996/01/01. PubMed PMID: 8532808.

[15] Momeni, A., Lee, G. K. A case of intraoperative venous congestion of the entire DIEP-flap--a novel salvage technique and review of the literature. *Microsurgery*. 2010;30(6):443-6. Epub. 2010/09/30. doi: 10.1002/micr.20774. PubMed PMID: 20878727.

[16] Pennington, D. G., Hassall, M. The free transverse rectus abdominis myocutaneous flap in breast reconstruction after mastectomy. *The Australian and New Zealand journal of surgery*. 1991;61(6):446-51. Epub. 1991/06/01. PubMed PMID: 1829352.

[17] Serafin, D., Voci, V. E., Georgiade, N. G. Microsurgical composite tissue transplantation: indications and technical considerations in breast reconstruction following mastectomy. *Plastic and reconstructive surgery*. 1982;70(1):24-36. Epub. 1982/07/01. PubMed PMID: 7089105.
[18] Kerr-Valentic, M. A., Gottlieb, L. J., Agarwal, J. P. The retrograde limb of the internal mammary vein: an additional outflow option in DIEP flap breast reconstruction. *Plastic and reconstructive surgery*. 2009;124(3): 717-21. Epub. 2009/09/05. doi: 10.1097/PRS.0b013e3181b179fc. Pub Med PMID: 19730291.
[19] Galanis, C., Nguyen, P., Koh, J., Roostaeian, J., Festekjian, J., Crisera, C. Microvascular lifeboats: a stepwise approach to intraoperative venous congestion in DIEP flap breast reconstruction. *Plastic and reconstructive surgery*. 2014;134(1):20-7. Epub. 2014/07/17. doi: 10.1097/PRS. 0000000000000271. PubMed PMID: 25028816.
[20] Li, S., Mu, L., Li, Y., Xu, J., Yang, M., Zhao, Z., et al. Breast reconstruction with the free bipedicled inferior TRAM flap by anastomosis to the proximal and distal ends of the internal mammary vessels. *Journal of reconstructive microsurgery*. 2002;18(3):161-8. Epub. 2002/05/15. doi: 10.1055/s-2002-28498. PubMed PMID: 120070 53.
[21] Schwabegger, A. H., Ninkovic, M. M., Moriggl, B., Waldenberger, P., Brenner, E., Wechselberger, G., et al. Internal mammary veins: classification and surgical use in free-tissue transfer. *Journal of reconstructive microsurgery*. 1997;13(1):17-23. Epub. 1997/01/01. doi: 10.1055/s-2008-1063936. PubMed PMID: 9120838.
[22] Mackey, S. P., Ramsey, K. W. Exploring the myth of the valveless internal mammary vein--a cadaveric study. *Journal of plastic, reconstructive and aesthetic surgery: JPRAS*. 2011;64(9):1174-9. Epub 2011/05/07. doi: 10.1016/j.bjps.2011.03.045. PubMed PMID: 21546327.
[23] Wagner, D. S., Michelow, B. J., Hartrampf, C. R., Jr. Double-pedicle TRAM flap for unilateral breast reconstruction. *Plastic and reconstructive surgery*. 1991;88(6):987-97. Epub. 1991/12/11. PubMed PMID: 1835103.
[24] Kroll, S. S., Schusterman, M. A., Reece, G. P., Miller, M. J., Robb, G., Evans, G. Abdominal wall strength, bulging, and hernia after TRAM flap breast reconstruction. *Plastic and reconstructive surgery*. 1995; 96 (3):616-9. Epub. 1995/09/01. PubMed PMID: 7638285.
[25] Harashina, T., Sone, K., Inoue, T., Fukuzumi, S., Enomoto, K. Augmentation of circulation of pedicled transverse rectus abdominis

musculocutaneous flaps by microvascular surgery. *British journal of plastic surgery*. 1987;40(4):367-70. Epub. 1987/07/01. PubMed PMID: 2957016.

[26] Takayanagi, S. Extended transverse rectus abdominis musculocutaneous flap. *Plastic and reconstructive surgery*. 1993;92(4):757-8. Epub. 1993/09/01. PubMed PMID: 8356140.

[27] Semple, J. L. Retrograde microvascular augmentation (turbocharging) of a single-pedicle TRAM flap through a deep inferior epigastric arterial and venous loop. *Plastic and reconstructive surgery*. 1994;93(1):109-17. Epub. 1994/01/01. PubMed PMID: 8278465.

[28] Arnez, Z. M., Scamp, T. The bipedicled free TRAM flap. *British journal of plastic surgery*. 1992;45(3):214-8. Epub. 1992/04/01. PubMed PMID: 1596662.

[29] Blondeel, P. N., Boeckx, W. D. Refinements in free flap breast reconstruction: the free bilateral deep inferior epigastric perforator flap anastomosed to the internal mammary artery. *British journal of plastic surgery*. 1994;47(7):495-501. Epub. 1994/10/01. PubMed PMID: 79528 20.

[30] Ng, R. L., Youssef, A., Kronowitz, S. J., Lipa, J. E., Potochny, J., Reece, G. P. Technical variations of the bipedicled TRAM flap in unilateral breast reconstruction: effects of conventional versus microsurgical techniques of pedicle transfer on complications rates. *Plastic and reconstructive surgery*. 2004;114(2):374-84; discussion 85-8. Epub. 2004/07/28. PubMed PMID: 15277802.

[31] Lejour, M., Dome, M. Abdominal wall function after rectus abdominis transfer. *Plastic and reconstructive surgery*. 1991;87(6):1054-68. Epub. 1991/06/01. PubMed PMID: 1827922.

[32] Berrino, P., Casabona, F., Adami, M., Muggianu, M. The "parasite" TRAM flap for autogenous tissue breast reconstruction in patients with vertical midabdominal scars. *Annals of plastic surgery*. 1999;43(2):119-26. Epub. 1999/08/24. PubMed PMID: 10454315.

[33] Ali, R. S., Garrido, A., Ramakrishnan, V. Stacked free hemi-DIEP flaps: a method of autologous breast reconstruction in a patient with midline abdominal scarring. *British journal of plastic surgery*. 2002;55(4):351-3. Epub. 2002/08/06. PubMed PMID: 12160543.

[34] Das-Gupta, R., Busic, V., Begic, A. Deep inferior epigastric perforator flap (DIEP) breast reconstruction in the presence of a midline vertical scar. *Journal of plastic, reconstructive and aesthetic surgery: JPRAS*. 2006;59(6):675-6. Epub. 2006/07/05. PubMed PMID: 16817262.

[35] Schoeller, T., Wechselberger, G., Roger, J., Hussl, H., Huemer, G. M. Management of infraumbilical vertical scars in DIEP-flaps by crossover anastomosis. *Journal of plastic, reconstructive and aesthetic surgery: JPRAS*. 2007;60(5):524-8. Epub. 2007/04/03. doi: 10.1016/j.bjps.2006.11.008. PubMed PMID: 17399662.

[36] Pennington, D. G., Nettle, W. J., Lam, P. Microvascular augmentation of the blood supply of the contralateral side of the free transverse rectus abdominis musculocutaneous flap. *Annals of plastic surgery*. 1993;31(2):123-6; discussion 6-7. Epub. 1993/08/01. PubMed PMID: 8215126.

[37] Lam, T. C., Sellars, G. D. Free perforator crossover TRAM flap for breast reconstruction. *Annals of plastic surgery*. 2003;50(2):126-31. Epub. 2003/02/05. doi: 10.1097/01.SAP.0000032307.61429.9E. PubMed PMID: 12567047.

[38] Rozen, W. M., Chubb, D., Grinsell, D., Ashton, M. W. The variability of the Superficial Inferior Epigastric Artery (SIEA) and its angiosome: A clinical anatomical study. *Microsurgery*. 2010;30(5):386-91. Epub. 2010/01/09. doi: 10.1002/micr.20750. PubMed PMID: 20058298.

[39] Hallock, G. G. Further clarification of the nomenclature for compound flaps. *Plastic and reconstructive surgery*. 2006;117(7):151e-60e. Epub. 2006/06/15. doi: 10.1097/01.prs.0000219178.20541.7f. PubMed PMID: 16772903.

[40] Rahn, D. D., Phelan, J. N., Roshanravan, S. M., White, A. B., Corton, M. M. Anterior abdominal wall nerve and vessel anatomy: clinical implications for gynecologic surgery. *American journal of obstetrics and gynecology*. 2010;202(3):234 e1-5. Epub. 2009/12/22. doi: 10.1016/j.ajog.2009.10.878. PubMed PMID: 20022582.

[41] Kisielinski, K., Conze, J., Murken, A. H., Lenzen, N. N., Klinge, U., Schumpelick, V. The Pfannenstiel or so called "bikini cut": still effective more than 100 years after first description. *Hernia: the journal of hernias and abdominal wall surgery*. 2004;8(3):177-81. Epub. 2004/03/05. doi: 10.1007/s10029-004-0210-0. PubMed PMID: 14997364.

[42] Parrett, B. M., Caterson, S. A., Tobias, A. M., Lee, B. T. DIEP flaps in women with abdominal scars: are complication rates affected? *Plastic and reconstructive surgery*. 2008;121(5):1527-31. Epub. 2008/05/06. doi: 10.1097/PRS.0b013e31816b14a5. PubMed PMID: 18453974.

[43] Taylor, G. I., Doyle, M., McCarten, G. The Doppler probe for planning flaps: anatomical study and clinical applications. *British journal of plastic surgery*. 1990;43(1):1-16. Epub. 1990/01/01. PubMed PMID: 2178717.

[44] Giunta, R. E., Geisweid, A., Feller, A. M. The value of preoperative Doppler sonography for planning free perforator flaps. *Plastic and reconstructive surgery*. 2000;105(7):2381-6. Epub. 2000/06/09. PubMed PMID: 10845290.

[45] Hallock, G. G. Doppler sonography and color duplex imaging for planning a perforator flap. *Clinics in plastic surgery*. 2003;30(3):347-57, v-vi. Epub. 2003/08/15. PubMed PMID: 12916592.

[46] Masia, J., Clavero, J. A., Larranaga, J. R., Alomar, X., Pons, G., Serret, P. Multidetector-row computed tomography in the planning of abdominal perforator flaps. *Journal of plastic, reconstructive and aesthetic surgery: JPRAS*. 2006;59(6):594-9. Epub. 2006/05/24. doi: 10. 1016/j.bjps.2005.10.024. PubMed PMID: 16716952.

[47] Masia, J., Larranaga, J., Clavero, J. A., Vives, L., Pons, G., Pons, J. M. The value of the multidetector row computed tomography for the preoperative planning of deep inferior epigastric artery perforator flap: our experience in 162 cases. *Annals of plastic surgery*. 2008;60(1):29-36. Epub. 2008/02/19. doi: 10.1097/SAP.0b013e31805003c2. PubMed PMID: 18281792.

[48] Uppal, R. S., Casaer, B., Van Landuyt, K., Blondeel, P. The efficacy of preoperative mapping of perforators in reducing operative times and complications in perforator flap breast reconstruction. *Journal of plastic, reconstructive and aesthetic surgery: JPRAS*. 2009;62(7):859-64. Epub. 2008/05/21. doi: 10.1016/j.bjps.2008.04.015. PubMed PMID: 18490207.

[49] Lee, G. K., Fox, P. M., Riboh, J., Hsu, C., Saber, S., Rubin, G. D., et al. Computed tomography angiography in microsurgery: indications, clinical utility, and pitfalls. *Eplasty*. 2013;13:e42. Epub. 2013/09/12. PubMed PMID: 24023972; PubMed Central PMCID: PMC3742152.

[50] Keys, K. A., Louie, O., Said, H. K., Neligan, P. C., Mathes, D. W. Clinical utility of CT angiography in DIEP breast reconstruction. *Journal of plastic, reconstructive and aesthetic surgery: JPRAS*. 2013;66 (3):e61-5. Epub. 2012/10/23. doi: 10.1016/j.bjps.2012.09.025. PubMed PMID: 23084649.

[51] Alonso-Burgos, A., Garcia-Tutor, E., Bastarrika, G., Benito, A., Dominguez, P. D., Zubieta, J. L. Preoperative planning of DIEP and SGAP flaps: preliminary experience with magnetic resonance angiography using 3-tesla equipment and blood-pool contrast medium. *Journal of plastic, reconstructive and aesthetic surgery: JPRAS*. 2010;63 (2):298-304. Epub. 2009/01/06. doi: 10.1016/j.bjps.2008.11.009. Pub Med PMID: 19121986.

[52] Newman, M. I., Samson, M. C., Tamburrino, J. F., Swartz, K. A., Brunworth, L. An investigation of the application of laser-assisted indocyanine green fluorescent dye angiography in pedicle transverse rectus abdominus myocutaneous breast reconstruction. *The Canadian journal of plastic surgery = Journal canadien de chirurgie plastique*. 2011;19(1):e1-5. Epub. 2012/03/02. PubMed PMID: 22379372; PubMed Central PMCID: PMC3086506.

[53] Desai, N. D., Miwa, S., Kodama, D., Koyama, T., Cohen, G., Pelletier, M. P., et al. A randomized comparison of intraoperative indocyanine green angiography and transit-time flow measurement to detect technical errors in coronary bypass grafts. *The Journal of thoracic and cardiovascular surgery*. 2006;132(3):585-94. Epub. 2006/08/29. doi: 10. 1016/j.jtcvs.2005.09.061. PubMed PMID: 16935114.

[54] Komorowska-Timek, E., Gurtner, G. C. Intraoperative perfusion mapping with laser-assisted indocyanine green imaging can predict and prevent complications in immediate breast reconstruction. *Plastic and reconstructive surgery*. 2010;125(4):1065-73. Epub. 2010/03/26. doi: 10.1097/PRS.0b013e3181d17f80. PubMed PMID: 20335859.

[55] Rubben, A., Eren, S., Krein, R., Younossi, H., Bohler, U., Wienert, V. Infrared videoangiofluorography of the skin with indocyanine green--rat random cutaneous flap model and results in man. *Microvascular research*. 1994;47(2):240-51. Epub. 1994/03/01. doi: 10.1006/mvre. 1994.1018. PubMed PMID: 8022322.

[56] Holm, C., Mayr, M., Hofter, E., Becker, A., Pfeiffer, U. J., Muhlbauer, W. Intraoperative evaluation of skin-flap viability using laser-induced fluorescence of indocyanine green. *British journal of plastic surgery*. 2002;55(8):635-44. Epub. 2003/01/29. PubMed PMID: 12550116.

[57] Holm, C., Tegeler, J., Mayr, M., Becker, A., Pfeiffer, U. J., Muhlbauer, W. Monitoring free flaps using laser-induced fluorescence of indocyanine green: a preliminary experience. *Microsurgery*. 2002;22(7): 278-87. Epub. 2002/10/31. doi: 10.1002/micr.10052. PubMed PMID: 12404345.

[58] Gurtner, G. C., Jones, G. E., Neligan, P. C., Newman, M. I., Phillips, B. T., Sacks, J. M., et al. Intraoperative laser angiography using the SPY system: review of the literature and recommendations for use. *Annals of surgical innovation and research*. 2013;7(1):1. Epub. 2013/01/08. doi: 10.1186/1750-1164-7-1. PubMed PMID: 23289664; PubMed Central PMCID: PMC3558356.

[59] Giunta, R. E., Holzbach, T., Taskov, C., Holm, P. S., Brill, T., Busch, R., et al. Prediction of flap necrosis with laser induced indocyanine green fluorescence in a rat model. *British journal of plastic surgery*. 2005;58(5):695-701. Epub. 2005/06/01. doi: 10.1016/j.bjps.2005.02.018. PubMed PMID: 15925341.

[60] Jallali, N., Ridha, H., Butler, P. E. Postoperative monitoring of free flaps in UK plastic surgery units. *Microsurgery*. 2005;25(6):469-72. Epub. 2005/09/01. doi: 10.1002/micr.20148. PubMed PMID: 16134095.

[61] Cody, H. S., 3rd, Urban, J. A. Internal mammary node status: a major prognosticator in axillary node-negative breast cancer. *Annals of surgical oncology*. 1995;2(1):32-7. Epub. 1995/01/01. PubMed PMID: 7834452.

[62] Veronesi, U., Marubini, E., Mariani, L., Valagussa, P., Zucali, R. The dissection of internal mammary nodes does not improve the survival of breast cancer patients. 30-year results of a randomised trial. *European journal of cancer*. 1999;35(9):1320-5. Epub. 2000/02/05. PubMed PMID: 10658521.

[63] Fitzgibbons, P. L., Page, D. L., Weaver, D., Thor, A. D., Allred, D. C., Clark, G. M., et al. Prognostic factors in breast cancer. College of American Pathologists Consensus Statement 1999. *Archives of pathology and laboratory medicine*. 2000;124(7):966-78. Epub. 2000/07/11. doi: 10.1043/0003-9985(2000)124<0966:PFIBC>2.0.CO;2. Pub Med PMID: 10888772.

[64] Ahmed, M., Purushotham, A. D., Douek, M. Novel techniques for sentinel lymph node biopsy in breast cancer: a systematic review. *The Lancet Oncology*. 2014;15(8):e351-62. Epub. 2014/07/06. doi: 10.1016/S1470-2045(13)70590-4. PubMed PMID: 24988938.

[65] Veronesi, U., Paganelli, G., Viale, G., Luini, A., Zurrida, S., Galimberti, V., et al. A randomized comparison of sentinel-node biopsy with routine axillary dissection in breast cancer. *The New England journal of medicine*. 2003;349(6):546-53. Epub. 2003/08/09. doi: 10.1056/NEJMoa012782. PubMed PMID: 12904519.

[66] Madsen, E., Gobardhan, P., Bongers, V., Albregts, M., Burgmans, J., De Hooge, P., et al. The impact on post-surgical treatment of sentinel lymph node biopsy of internal mammary lymph nodes in patients with breast cancer. *Annals of surgical oncology*. 2007;14(4):1486-92. Epub. 2007/01/27. doi: 10.1245/s10434-006-9230-6. PubMed PMID: 17253106; PubMed Central PMCID: PMC1914262.

[67] Leidenius, M. H., Krogerus, L. A., Toivonen, T. S., Leppanen, E. A., von Smitten, K. A. The clinical value of parasternal sentinel node biopsy in breast cancer. *Annals of surgical oncology*. 2006;13(3):321-6. Epub. 2006/02/18. doi: 10.1245/ASO.2006.02.022. PubMed PMID: 16485152.

[68] Kong, A. L., Tereffe, W., Hunt, K. K., Yi, M., Kang, T., Weatherspoon, K., et al. Impact of internal mammary lymph node drainage identified by preoperative lymphoscintigraphy on outcomes in patients with stage I to III breast cancer. *Cancer*. 2012;118(24):6287-96. Epub. 2012/06/01. doi: 10.1002/cncr.27564. PubMed PMID: 22648744; PubMed Central PMCID: PMC3913471.

In: Advances in Surgical Procedures
Editor: Miriam Figueroa
ISBN: 978-1-63482-461-3

Chapter 5

Advances in Surgical Procedures Thyroid Goitres: Surgery for Large and Difficult Goitres

Yassar A. Qureshi, MBBS, MRCS, MSc
and Fiona McClenaghan, BSc, MBBS
The Royal London Hospital, London, UK

Abstract

Thyroidectomy for goitres can often be challenging, but this is especially apparent for large and difficult goitres. These can often reach very large sizes prior to surgical intervention, and may also extend into, and adhere to, surrounding structures. This makes the surgery more exigent, and increases the risk of damaging major structures inadvertently, including the recurrent laryngeal nerve and parathyroid glands. In this chapter, we describe the optimal pre-operative management, including essential imaging to assess the thyroid, and investigations necessary for careful operative planning. We describe the operation for such glands in a logical manner, and incorporate techniques and advances which make the surgery more straightforward, and allow the surgeon to carefully identify and preserve vital structures. Further, we describe how to approach specific complications resulting from surgery for large goitres, including both intra-operative techniques and post-operative care.

Introduction

"Can the thyroid in the state of enlargement be removed? Emphatically, experience answers no… every stroke of the knife will be followed by a torrent of blood and lucky if his victims lived long enough for him to finish his horrid butchery! No honest and sensible surgeon would ever engage in it."

Samuel Gross, 1866

This famous quote by Samuel Gross, a US surgeon is, thankfully, rarely the case in contemporary thyroid surgery. However, the thyroid surgeon can certainly appreciate his exasperation at this form of surgery, owing to the very high risk and demanding nature of the operation. His particular reference to an enlarged thyroid gland, or goitre, makes it a more remarkable observation, as thyroid surgery for such a diseased thyroid is much more challenging and carries its own peculiar and significant risks.

The ancient Chinese first described large goitres as early as 2700 BC, but it was not until much later that the disease was understood. The Romans coined the term goitre, from the Latin 'gutter' or throat, and indeed, it was Julius Caesar who observed that goitres tended to be endemic in his conquered Gauls- a fact owing to the low iodine concentration in the local water.

Although herbal remedies, incantations and exorcisms were used not uncommonly for the treatment of goitres, surgery was first described in 952 AD. Ali Ibn Abbas, an Arab Physician, performed a successful excision of a goitre under opium sedation. In the 12th Century in Italy, surgeons continued to perform this operation, albeit with an incredibly high mortality rate. It was not until 1791 that a French Surgeon, Pierre Joseph Desault, refined the surgery, with some success, but mortality remained so high that the French Academy of Medicine took the drastic action of banning the operation in 1850. With future developments in the field of anaesthesia, antisepsis and surgical technology, the operation resumed, with improved outcomes. Although the words of Samuel Gross held true at the time, it should not be forgotten that the first Surgeon to achieve a Nobel Prize was Theodore Kocher, for his work on thyroid physiology and refinement of surgical technique for the goitre.

Surgery for large goitres can be challenging. Goitres may reach very large sizes, and will invariably, to some degree, distort anatomy, thus making dissection in correct tissue planes problematic. Vital structures may be more difficult to identify, making the risk of complications more pronounced.

Furthermore, the sheer size of the goitre often means the surgery is longer, with more dissection than anticipated, and the goitres may encroach into seldom visited body cavities, such as the chest.

Careful operative planning and investigation is most useful in ensuring that an optimal operation is performed. Exposure is key to good dissection, and thus certain intra-operative techniques may allow better access to tissue planes. After such operations, the patient is, perhaps, more likely to suffer post-operative complications and protracted recovery, and so must be carefully monitored and reassessed, to ensure their good recovery and early discharge.

Pre-Operative Planning

Examination

A thorough examination of the patient should be performed by the operating surgeon. This is to ascertain the size of the goitre, and plan for the site of the incision to give optimal access. Large thyroid glands may be due to benign or malignant disease. This needs to be ascertained pre-operatively, often by a combination of radiological and histopathological investigations. The importance of delineating the diagnosis prior to the operation is because malignant disease may require more extensive surgery to obtain clear margins, and may be associated with extended lymph node dissection. Although true for inflammatory disease too, malignant disease is often invasive into surrounding structures. Tissue planes may be disrupted and dissection more difficult. Indeed, if a sub-total or debulking operation is envisaged, for example to relieve compression of the airway, this should be determined pre-operatively, rather than in the midst of the operation.

On examination, local lymphadenopathy should be assessed for, and previous scars should be specifically looked for. In some cases, a re-do operation will need to be performed, which are typically more challenging, and previous scars will need to be incorporated into the new incision. This is to ensure both good access, but also a reasonable cosmetic outcome for the patient.

Ideally, if possible, it is better to operate on euthyroid patients, and hence a pre-operative review by an endocrinologist is beneficial. This will minimise peri-operative erratic thyroid function, and avoid a potential 'thyroid storm' during the operation. Calcium levels should also be checked to ensure normal parathyroid function. The vocal cords and voice quality should be checked independently, and the results documented. This is especially important given that 1% of the population will have a unilateral asymptomatic paralysis of the cord. Medical co-morbidity should be assessed and optimised, to ensure minimal peri-operative risk, and to enhance healing and recovery.

Radiological Investigation

Most patients presenting with thyroid problems will undergo an ultrasound scan as an initial radiological investigation. This will give an indication as to the size of the thyroid goitre, and its relationship to surrounding structures. However, if dealing with large goitres, a contrast enhanced computerised tomography (CT) scan is especially useful, as it will give significantly more detailed information regarding the dimensions of the thyroid. In, particular, it will also clearly show the proximity to surrounding vital structures, and show extension of the thyroid gland into the retrosternal space or the thoracic cavity. These factors will allow the surgeon to carefully plan for the operation, not only in terms of the incision, but also the best method to approach the dissection of the gland. Consistent landmarks such as the trachea and carotid sheath can be helpful to convey the radiological findings to the actual dissection. However, more slender structures such as the recurrent laryngeal nerve and parathyroid glands will not be seen radiologically; in the case of the latter, unless there is a concurrent parathyroid adenoma. A magnetic resonance imaging (MRI) scan provides similar detail to the CT scanning, and is preferred in some units.

Previous radiotherapy to the neck can cause tissue damage by inflammation and necrosis and even if surgery is many years later, tissue planes will be compromised, anatomy may be distorted, and healing may be protracted.

Anaesthetic Review

The anaesthetist should be familiar with difficult and shared airways, and review the patient prior to the operation. This is to familiarise oneself with the patient's medical history, biochemical thyroid status and to perform an examination. Particular history of airway and respiratory disease should be elucidated, and any possibility of airway encroachment explored. The patient's oropharynx should be thoroughly assessed: this will allow better planning for anaesthesia and intubation. Any potential disease involvement of the trachea must be fully explored, as it should be borne in mind that longstanding involvement of the trachea by a goitre may be associated with tracheomalacia. Positional breathlessness, dysphagia, and stridor should be evaluated, if present. Rarely, a very large or retrosternal goitre may compress the superior vena cava.

For thyroid surgery, owing to the ever-present risks to the airway, a definitive airway for the extent of surgery should be performed. This would normally involve a cuffed endotracheal tube. Fibre-optic intubation may be useful in cases where there is some degree of airway obstruction. Indeed, a pre-operative tracheostomy may be required where complete airway obstruction is imminent. There is no specific guideline on the use of paralytic agents, but it may help in reducing laryngeal reflexes. A strong analgesic, such as remifentanyl, is often used, as apart from its analgesic effect, it contributes to a mild hypotension, thus aiding the minimisation of blood loss. Dexamethasone at induction may also contribute to reduced inflammation and oedema around the airway and dissection field.

Intraoperative Technique for Goitre Surgery

The normal thyroid gland lies at the anterior aspect of the neck. It has two lobes, normally about 5cm each in size, connected by a central isthmus overlying the trachea. Generally, the superior aspects of the lobes are narrow, and become broader inferiorly. Medially, the relations of each lobe are the larynx, trachea and oesophagus, anterolaterally the strap muscles and the sternocleidomastoid and posteriorly the carotid sheath. These relations are important to bear in mind when approaching a large thyroid. The gland itself is surrounded by a thin fibrous capsule, which extends over the trachea (the pre-trachea fascia) and laterally onto the carotid sheath. When a large goitre is encountered, it often extends laterally, displacing the carotid sheath, but if the goitre is secondary to an invasive disease, it may infiltrate into any surrounding structure.

Initial Operative Approach

The patient is positioned supine on the operative table, with the head in extension, which can be achieved by placing sand bags beneath the shoulders. The head is placed on a circular head ring, and the anaesthetist should ensure that they are content with the endotracheal tube positioning prior to the preparation and draping of the patient. Once an unencumbered sterile field is set up, the surgeon can mark the skin incision. This usually lies 2-3cms above the sternal notch, ideally in a skin crease. However, the exact site and extent of the skin incision may vary dependent on the size of the thyroid. Indeed, if a re-do operation is being performed, the old scar should be incorporated into the contemporary incision.

Once the skin and platysma is breached, the anterior jugular veins will be encountered, and if they are obscuring the operative field, can be ligated. Once flaps are raised, the infrahyoid muscles are delineated, separated in the midline and the central portion of the thyroid gland exposed. The strap muscles are dissected off the thyroid lobes. This will expose the superior pole of the thyroid, which should be dissected off surrounding structures in the correct plane beneath its capsule. The dissection is within the sterno-laryngeal (or Joll's) triangle, constituting the midline, infrahyoid muscles and the superior thyroid pedicle. Once the superior pole and its vascular pedicle are secured, the remainder of the thyroid can be mobilised, and the inferior thyroid pole approached. The middle thyroid vein, draining into the internal jugular vein, should be identified and ligated, prior to inadvertent avulsion.

Anterolateral Dissection

The strap muscles form this relationship with the thyroid, and the surgeon will encounter first the sternothyroid, then the sternohyoid and the superior belly of the omohyoid. The pairs of strap muscles converge in the midline and separated to gain access to the thyroid gland. Division of these muscles may ease access in dissecting the superior lobe of the thyroid. It can be safely performed by dividing the sternothyroid and sternohyoid muscles transversely as close to their origin in the midline as possible, as the specific branches of the ansa cervicalis which innervate these muscles approach from inferiorly. The divided muscles can then be retracted superior-laterally to expose the large superior pole of the thyroid. After excision of the gland, continuity of the muscle edges can be restored using interrupted sutures.

Often, between the sternothyroid and sternohyoid muscles, there lies an avascular plane, dissection through which will enable the surgeon to reach the carotid sheath. Development of this plane may be sufficient to allow the superior pole to be safely mobilised. Indeed, the deeper sternothyroid may still be transected, but division of the sternohyoid can be altogether avoided.

When approaching the superior lobe where there is clear invasion into or toward the muscles, the surgeon can employ the 'back door to thyoid' approach. This involves dissection of the sternocleidomastoid off the strap muscles. A plane between the carotid sheath and the lateral aspect of the sternohyoid is then developed, which allows access to the thyroid gland. If required, the inferior belly of the omohyoid may be transected to allow further access. This technique allows access to the lateral aspect of the thyroid for dissection, and can aid the avoidance of a protracted and bloody dissection if there is thyroid invasion or encroachment laterally, as may be found in very large goitres, goitres secondary to malignancy or in recurrent multinodular goitre.

Posterior Dissection and the Parathyroid Glands

The large goitre tends to enlarge in this direction, and can push the carotid sheath from a posterior to a lateral relation. The carotid sheath transmits the common carotid artery, and laterally the internal jugular vein, with the vagus nerve lying in between. The ansa cervicalis, motor nerves which innervate ipsilateral strap muscles, lie anteriorly on the sheath.

As mentioned, dissection of the plane between the medial sheath and the thyroid aids the mobilisation of the large thyroid. Owing to the potential catastrophe of injury to the carotid sheath structures, dissection around this relation should be slow and careful. If thyroid disease is invading onto the sheath, then the sheath can be carefully dissected off immediately above the underlying vessels.

The parathyroid glands, two superior and two inferior, will also be encountered during posterior dissection of the thyroid. The position of the parathyroid glands is not always consistent, and they may be located either outside or within the thyroid capsule, or in 0.2% of cases deep within the thyroid parenchyma.[1] The superior parathyroid glands, which arise from the fourth branchial pouch, are more consistently located, with most posterior to the superior thyroid pole. The inferior glands, arising from the third pouch, are often more variably located, but generally should lie around the lower thyroid pole. Normal parathyroid glands are only 5mm in size and often difficult to identify, particularly in a bloody dissection field. However, their identification and preservation is of utmost importance in good surgical practise. Interestingly, even with very large goitres, the non-ectopic parathyroid glands are consistently located within the expected field of variation. Pre-operatively, parathyroid glands, unless aberrantly large, will seldom be seen on ultrasonography or cross-sectional imaging.

The superior parathyroid glands lie superior to the inferior thyroid artery, on the posterolateral aspect of the thyroid gland. When dissecting the pre-tracheal fascia off the thyroid from a lateral to medial direction, the superior parathyroids will become apparent, and will most often lie deep to the recurrent laryngeal nerve.

The inferior parathyroid glands lie below the inferior thyroid artery, and are generally more anterior than the recurrent laryngeal nerve. Again, when dissecting the inferior pole of the thyroid, these will become apparent as the surgeon comes from lateral to medial, whilst the thyroid is lifted to visualise its posterior aspect.[1,2]

Rather than inadvertent excision, the more common cause of parathyroid function failure after thyroid surgery is the devascularisation of the parathyroid glands. This can easily be caused by rough dissection, inadequate field of vision, or mass ligature of vessels. In 80% of cases, the parathyroids will receive an arterial blood supply from branches originating from the inferior thyroid artery. Regardless of the size of the goitre, this pivotal vessel and its immediate surroundings should be clearly visualised. To avoid devascularisation of the parathyroids, rather than ligate the main trunk of the inferior thyroid artery, only its terminal branches on the pre-tracheal fascia of the thyroid capsule should be ligated. This will ensure reasonable blood supply to the parathyroid glands and avoid post-operative hypocalcaemia. In the circumstance where the parathyroid glands are embedded within the thyroid parenchyma, a peri-capsular dissection can be performed, whereby a cuff of thyroid tissue is left attached to parathyroid to avoid vascular injury to the parathyroid gland.

In absolutely unavoidable situations, if the parathyroids are not all accounted for prior to excision of the thyroid gland, then the specimen must be examined.

The parathyroid glands, if salvageable, can be cut into small pieces and implanted into a small pocket fashioned in the sternocleidomastoid muscle.

This scenario may be encountered, for example, when performing a curative resection for malignant disease which is infiltrating into or around the parathyroid glands.

Medial Dissection and the Recurrent Laryngeal Nerve

Medially, the surgeon will encounter the larynx and trachea. The thyroid goitre which is applied to these structures can be gently dissected off. If there is invasion into the trachea, then a small cuff may be excised with a primary suture repair performed, but dissecting into the larynx is more haphazard owing to the presence of the vocal cords and their nerves. Dissection must remain on the thyroid capsule at this border, and must only be conducted once the recurrent laryngeal nerves and the parathyroid glands have been clearly identified: this is perhaps the most crucial part of a thyroidectomy.

The external laryngeal nerve is a branch of the superior laryngeal nerve, which in turns originates from the vagus. It innervates the cricothyroid muscle, damage to which affects the quality and tonality of phonation. It lies anterior and medial to the superior thyroid artery, although in 20% of people it is intertwined within branches of the artery.[3] It is thus necessary that the superior pole of the thyroid is dissected completely free and the superior thyroid vascular pedicle appropriately visualised. For large goitres, as mentioned previously, transection of the strap muscles, particularly the sternothyroid, would aid in obtaining access to the superior pole of the thyroid. Further, the ligation of the superior thyroid artery should be precise, to ensure that the nerve is not inadvertently divided.

The most critical aspect of a thyroidectomy, made more difficult by large goitres, is the identification and preservation of the recurrent laryngeal nerve. Its inadvertent iatrogenic injury will have significant impact on the patient's quality of life; indeed, bilateral injury to the nerve can be life-threatening. Knowledge of the anatomy of the nerve is paramount, including its aberrations: indeed, the right and left recurrent laryngeal nerves run a different course. At the root of the neck, the right vagus gives off its right recurrent laryngeal branch. It winds around the subclavian artery and emerges behind the common carotid artery. Here, it takes a medial course and enters the right trachea-oesophageal groove. The left recurrent laryngeal nerve originates from the left vagus just lateral to the aortic arch, which it winds around to emerge medially into the left trachea-oesophageal groove. Once in the groove, the nerves ascend and pass either through or behind the ligament of Berry and into the larynx. This ligament is where the pre-tracheal fascia condenses between the thyroid and the anteromedial trachea.[3,4] Division or ligation of the ligament here will undoubtedly injure the nerves. Care must be taken when dissecting the superior pole of the thyroid around the cricothyroid muscle, where either inadvertent damage to the ligament of Berry, nerve, or the muscle itself, can affect vocal cord function.

The inferior thyroid artery provides a most useful landmark when identifying the nerve. Although the exact relationship between the two is not always consistent, they can be identified in the same vicinity. The nerve can run superficial to the artery (25% of patients), deep (50%) or intertwined between branches of the artery (25%).[4] The inferior pole of the thyroid is usually approached after the superior pole: anterior displacement of the superior lobe should give a clear view of the inferior pole, and dissection approached carefully from lateral to medial. Gentle lateral retraction of the carotid sheath will aid in exposure of the tissue planes where the nerve is located. Once the artery has been identified, with its pulsation, careful examination will reveal the nerve. This should be traced along its length all the way into the larynx. It should be dissected free with as minimal contact as possible in order to avoid neuropraxia. Ligation of the inferior thyroid artery should be of its terminal branches, precisely and one at a time.

The incidence of a right non-recurrent laryngeal nerve is up to 0.7% of the population. Here, the nerve directly enters the larynx coming from behind the common carotid artery. Non-recurrent laryngeal nerves are much rarer on the left, affecting 0.04% of patients. Of further note, although the nerves lie in the trachea-oesophageal groove in 80% of patients, they may traverse in and out of the groove, or may be lying outside of it.[4] Hence, medial dissection of the thyroid off the trachea must be deferred until the nerve is elucidated for its entire course.

Very rarely, when performing surgery for large goitres, malignant disease, or where a re-operation is performed, there may be an anticipation of disease involving the recurrent laryngeal nerve. For example, the nerve may be infiltrated by disease, making it impossible to dissect. This needs to be carefully discussed with the patient pre-operatively; the consideration of sacrifice of the nerve for disease control is a decision to be made jointly by the surgeon and the patient. The latter should be made fully aware of the possible implications on their quality of life following such an intervention.

Intra-operative nerve monitoring is not yet mandatory, but many surgeons do utilise it. If used, it must be borne in mind that it is not a substitute for actual visualisation of the nerve in its anticipated anatomical location. Further, false readings may be apparent if there is an effect on the nerve from local anaesthesia or from a neuromuscular blockade from an agent administered by the anaesthetist. Indeed, the tracheal-laryngeal electrode may become displaced, giving a false-negative reading. However, if used appropriately, it can audibly confirm gross nerve continuity, but should still be used in conjunction with correct anatomical correlation.

Although the recurrent laryngeal nerve provides the surgeon with some degree of anxiety, careful dissection, avoidance of mass ligature, and a detailed knowledge of nerve anatomy is sufficient to avoid inadvertent injury. Surgery for large goitres can make anatomical identification more challenging, but if key principles are carefully adhered to, the nerve should not be at risk. Meticulous dissection of the thyroid lobes, in a bloodless field and in the correct planes, will allow the surgeon to encounter the nerves, and the parathyroid glands, with a clear view.

Retrosternal Goitre

Although first described in 1749 by Albrecht von Haller, the famous Swiss anatomist, the precise definition of a retrosternal goitre remains debated. Generally, however, it is taken to mean where greater than 50% of the thyroid mass lay in the mediastinum, or below the thoracic inlet. This may be an extension from a normally located cervical goitre, or more rarely an ectopically sited thyroid gland which grows *de novo*. The incidence varies geographically, ranging from between 2-19% of all thyroidectomies.[5,6] The treatment for retrosternal goitre is extremely challenging, fraught with risk, and controversial; it most certainly is a distinct operation to a cervical thyroidectomy. We will briefly highlight some important points for this type of goitre.

The main clinical implications of retrosternal goitre are related to the pressure they exert on mediastinal structures. This can be primarily by the thyroid parenchyma itself, or from secondary events such as haemorrhage or malignant growth.

The common structures that are affected include the trachea and bronchus, oesophagus, the aortic arch, carotid artery and superior vena cava. In some instances, the goitre may extend over the pericardium and below the right atrium. Pre-operative planning with cross-sectional imaging is mandatory. The structures affected by the goitre need to be known prior to an operation, and if necessary, the aid of a cardiothoracic surgeon enlisted.

The approach to such goitres is mostly through a cervical incision, especially if they are relatively small, or only enter the very proximal mediastinum. If more extensive, then a partial or total median sternotomy (to the 4th intercostal space) is required.[6] This is particularly true if the goitre is abutting major vascular structures where there is a high risk of haemorrhage, if the goitre is largely positioned in the posterior mediastinum, or if the goitre is secondary to malignant disease.

The key phases of the operation, once the thyroid is exposed, is to ensure vascular control. This is true for the superior thyroid vessels, which can be safely ligated, but principally for larger vessels, such as the carotids or those around the aortic arch: proximal and distal control is advocated. This ensures that, in case of vascular injury, haemorrhage can be curtailed swiftly, and it also allows more confident dissection of the thyroid off these major vessels. The inferior thyroid vessels will still be located cervically, and the same principles as a standard thyroidectomy apply: care to avoid inadvertent injury to the recurrent laryngeal nerve, the careful ligation of its distal branches to avoid parathyroid gland devascularisation, and to carefully identify these structures prior to pursuing medial dissection. Where airway structures are involved by goitre, the anaesthetist must be kept fully alerted: if necessary, endobronchial ventilation instituted. Dissection of the gland is performed from superior to lateral to inferior, all the while applying gentle traction to help deliver the retrosternal portion of the gland into the wound.

The risks of a standard thyroidectomy, particularly parathyroid or recurrent laryngeal nerve injury, are magnified. This is sometimes because these structures are stretched or splayed into aberrant positions. Thus, the surgeon must very clearly identify these structures, moving to more normal anatomy and tracing them if necessary. It should be borne in mind that a torrential haemorrhage from the chest will unlikely be controlled by a cervical incision, and a sternotomy would thence be required. Patients, therefore, should be appropriately consented and fully informed of such risks.[6]

Lymph Node Dissection

For goitre secondary to malignancy, a lymph node harvest is advocated for both therapeutic and prognostic and staging purposes. Pre-operative assessment with MRI or Ultrasound Scanning is essential to be able to ascertain the degree of lymph node excision required.

Level VI neck dissection is most often performed for malignant disease, and such a harvest is aided by finding the recurrent laryngeal nerve in the low or mid-level of neck. It can then be traced superiorly, and the lymph nodes excised without jeopardising it. The thymus is included in the excision specimen, if possible. Lateral neck dissection tends to be more straightforward, unless there is invasion into the carotid sheath. Level IV dissection should be performed with care, as the thoracic duct may be injured, particularly if the nodes are affected by disease, and thus will be adherent.[7]

In some centres, sentinel lymph node biopsy has been performed for some thyroid cancers, but as yet there is no suggestion of enhanced outcome or improved staging information gleaned from this procedure. Indeed, misplacement of blue dye may cause spread of the stain across the whole operating field, making dissection trickier!

Post-Operative Care

The post-operative patient should, ideally, be nursed in area of direct observation, such as a high dependency unit at a 45 degree angle. Owing to the anatomical location of the thyroid and the field of dissection, airway compromise is an ever present threat, and should be specifically assessed for periodically.

Once the thyroid goitre is excised, prior to layered closure of the wound, a check and then re-check should be made to ensure haemostasis. A large expanding haematoma collecting in the wound can definitely cause airway compromise and is a surgical emergency. The thyroid is a very vascular organ, and bleeding should be controlled during the operation with precise suture ligation, clips or diathermy.

At the end, the entire bed should be thoroughly assessed, using warm saline wash, to review and address any bleeding. Positioning the patient in the head-down position will aid in this. Furthermore, the anaesthetist can be asked to induce several val salva manoeuvres, which may highlight further bleeding. If there is a tear in the thyroid capsule during dissection of the goitre, then this should be repaired with a fine suture, to control bleeding and also to stop the dissemination of thyroid cells. A bloody operative field makes thyroid surgery far more difficult, especially around the nerves and parathyroid glands, in this quintessential plane based operation. Larger vessels, such as the common carotid or internal jugular very rarely are involved with disease. If encountered, dissection must be performed with great care, to avoid a potentially catastrophic haemorrhage, and to avoid post-operative neurological complications.

The assistance of a vascular surgeon should be enlisted if there is any concern. Finally, prior to closure, a vacuum based drain (such as a Redivac®) may be left *in situ*, both to stop compression of the airway from a potential haematoma or inflammatory fluid, but also in order to monitor blood output in case of a large bleed.

If a haematoma does develop post-operatively, with airway compromise, then the wound and deeper sutures should be immediately removed to allow the haematoma to escape. Re-bleeding should warrant an early re-exploration of the wound, and any bleeding points addressed. Often, there is no active bleeding found, but rather generalised ooze. In this instance, a haemostatic adjunct, such as Surgicel®, may be used. A vacuum based drain should be left in the wound after a re-operation for bleeding.

It is mandatory for the surgeon and his or her equipment to remain sterile until the patient is successfully extubated. This is in case of immediate airway compromise where an emergency tracheostomy may be required. Bilateral injury to the recurrent laryngeal nerve will cause such an airway compromise, but thankfully, this is very rare indeed. More common is a neuropraxia, and this would be diagnosed if the surgeon had clearly delineated and ensured continuity of the nerves at the time of the operation. An elective tracheostomy is rarely required, unless there is very significant stenosis of the trachea. In the authors' experience, tracheomalacia is very rare, even after surgery for very large and longstanding goitres, and can be treated with a tracheal stent, rather than with a tracheostomy.

Unilateral recurrent laryngeal nerve injury or neuropraxia will cause a change or hoarseness in voice. A naso-endoscope should be performed to assess the vocal cords; neuropraxia will generally settle within a few weeks. If dysfunction persists, then early referral to a speech and language therapist may be of benefit. Of course, the patient should be fully counselled about the likely long-term effects of such an injury.

In the post-operative period, metabolic imbalances should be assessed for regularly, both clinically and by serum biochemical analysis. If a total thyroidectomy has been performed, then oral thyroxine is commenced, and serum concentrations monitored to ascertain the optimal dose. Serum calcium should be monitored regularly in the post-operative setting, as levels can fluctuate. At its worst, an imbalance in calcium homeostasis can cause cardiac dysfunction and arrest. Hypocalcaemia may be due to inadvertent excision of the parathyroid gland(s) or desvalcularisation.

For the latter cause, levels may improve over time. There is no set guideline on replacing calcium; rather this is based on local or even surgeon specific practise. Some centres place patients on calcium supplements pre-operatively. Most, however, will discharge patients after the operation on a short course of oral calcium supplements, regardless of the serum calcium or parathyroid hormone concentration. These serum analyses are continued in the outpatient setting until there is a consistent return to normal readings. If this is not achieved, then it may indicate permanent injury (after 6 months from surgery) to the parathyroid glands, and long-term replacement therapy is instituted. Intravenous calcium replacement is rarely required, and should be reserved for patients who either have a drastic drop in serum calcium concentration, or those who are symptomatic of hypocalcaemia.

Conclusion

Thyroid surgery for large goitres can be challenging, difficult and fraught with an increased risk of complications. However, it is this group of patients with thyroid disease- benign or malignant – who have large goitres that cause the most symptoms. Thus, they stand to benefit the most from surgical intervention. Detailed anatomical knowledge and adherence to safe dissection principles, along with some specific manoeuvres to improve access and visibility of the operative field, can render such operations a safe undertaking. Indeed, the surgeon, if competent and safe, may begin to enjoy these stimulating operations and the benefit the patient derives from them.

References

[1] Bailey B J, Calhoun K H, Friedman N R: Thyroid and Parathyroid. Atlas of Head and Neck Surgery – Otolaryngology, Bailey B J, Calhoun K H (Eds) 2nd Edition. Lippincott Williams and Wilkins (2001)

[2] Bliss R D, Gauger P C & Delbridge L W: Surgeon's approach to the Thyroid gland: surgical anatomy and the importance of technique. *World J. Surg.,* 2000; 24(8): 891 – 897.

[3] Randolph G.W : Surgical anatomy of the recurrent laryngeal nerve. Surgery of the thyroid and parathyroid glands; Randolph G W (Ed). Saunders, Philadelphia (2003)

[4] Gavilan J, Gavilan C. Recurrent laryngeal Nerve: Identification during thyroid and parathyroid surgery. *Arch Otolaryngol Head Neck Surg.,* 1986; 112: 1286 – 1288.

[5] Wheeler MH. Clinical Dilemma: Retrosternal Goitre. *Br. J. Surg.,* 1999; 87(4): 1235-6.

[6] Wheeler MH. The Surgical management of Retrosternal (Intrathorcic) Goiter. *World J. Endooc. Surg.,* 2013; 5(1): 28-30.

[7] Upile T, Jerjes W, Mahil J, *et al.* How to do it: The Difficult Thyroid. *Head Neck Oncol.,* 2011; 3: 54.

In: Advances in Surgical Procedures
Editor: Miriam Figueroa
ISBN: 978-1-63482-461-3

Chapter 6

Minimally Invasive Midface Lift Using Absorbable Sutures with Cones: A Step by Step Procedure

M. Goisis, A. Di Petrillo, L. Rosset, A. Kunderfranco, S. Mele, E. Stella and S. Khabouri

Abstract

Background: Since the invention of the first barbed (short) suture by Sulamanidze in the late 1990s, facial soft tissue lifting with subdermal sutures has a significant attraction for physician and patient alike. This study aimed to describe the authors' experience and the office techniques they have adopted to counteract the descent and laxity of facial soft tissues.

Methods: A retrospective chart review was performed during a period of 15 Months, from March 2013 to June 2014. The procedure was performed in 131 patients under local anesthesia using 2-0 absorbable polylactic sutures with 4 polylactic cones in their distal section (Silhouette Lift, Irvine, California).

The face was marked preoperatively to determine the appropriate vector of the thread and its two end exit points. The results were assessed objectively using serial photography with Canfield Camera System and subjectively according to patient assessment. Complications also were recorded.

Results: All but two patients were satisfied with the outcomes after treatment. Consensus ratings by two independent surgeons found that objective outcomes were divided among "excellent," "good," and "fair." The postoperative course was uneventful except for two patients who presented with major hematoma and another patient who had minor skin dimpling. These three complicated cases were resolved spontaneously without any surgical interventions.

Conclusion: The advantages of this technique are its simplicity, the fact that it produces no traumatic effects, and the fact that it can be performed with local anesthetic, reducing surgical time over current approaches.

Introduction

The process of facial aging involves all the layers of tissues. A general loss of volume is observed in the extracellular matrix of connective tissues, due to reduced synthesis of glicosaminoglicans and hyaluronic acid. Furthermore, alterations in the ultra structure of collagen and elastin lead to reduction of elasticity and increase of sagginess of soft tissues. The hypotrophy typical of the aging face and neck is then a process involving not only the skin but even fatty tissue and muscle.

The intermittent use of resorbable cone or barbed wires is aimed at preventing and treating the tissue sagginess and reinforcing the soft tissue of the face. The suture suspension technique falls in between the more aggressive and invasive procedures (for example, face lift) and the less invasive ones (such as fillers or Botox); the permanency of the results could measure up to 2 years. Coned and barbed wires allows accurate facial tissue repositioning by exerting immediate traction. Furthermore an even stronger force contrasting gravitational pull is provided by new collagen fibers formation. Starting around 2 months after the placement of the wires, the process of wire resorption leads to synthesis of collagen all around the wire, enhancing the traction over the tissues. The initial traction is produced by the presence of the slow-absorbing cones or barbs, which are reinforced by the buildup of new collagen formation. After the cones or barbs are reabsorbed the tissue traction is maintained by the collagen around and inside a series of knots interpolated along the wires. Further applications of wires on the same area are possible to enhance the support over soft tissue.

Methods

A retrospective chart review was performed during a period of 15 Months, from March 2013 to June 2014. The procedure was performed in 131 patients under local anesthesia using 2-0 absorbable polylactic sutures with 4 polylactic cones in their distal section (Silhouette Lift, Irvine, California).

61 patients underwent coned wires lift on the cheeks for correction of medium and low facial sagginess; 12 patients underwent wire lift in the eyebrow and frontal region; 29 patients underwent lift of the cervical region; 29 patients underwent coned wires lift in both the facial and cervical area.

The face was marked preoperatively to determine the appropriate vector of the thread and its two end exit points. The results were assessed objectively using serial photography with Canfield Camera System and subjectively according to patient assessment. Complications also were recorded.

The patients have been asked to give us an anonymous written feedback regarding the short term results with a simple scale by choosing among: very good, good, fair, bad, very bad.

For each patient pre and postoperative photos were sent to two independent surgeons to evaluate the aesthetic outcome. Results could be rated by a single scale marking among: very good, good, bad, very bad.

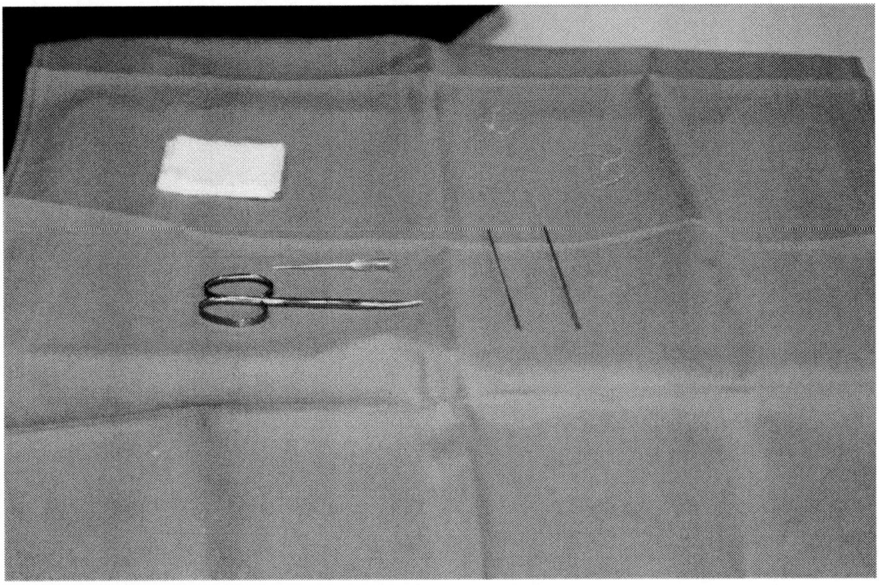

A: Materials (1): Coned wires, 18 G needle, scissors, bandages.

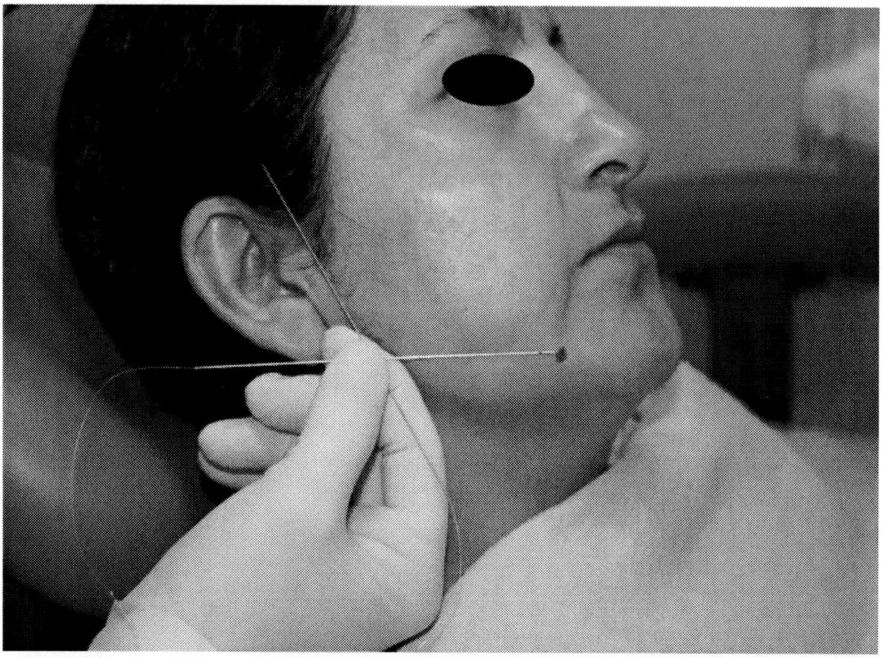

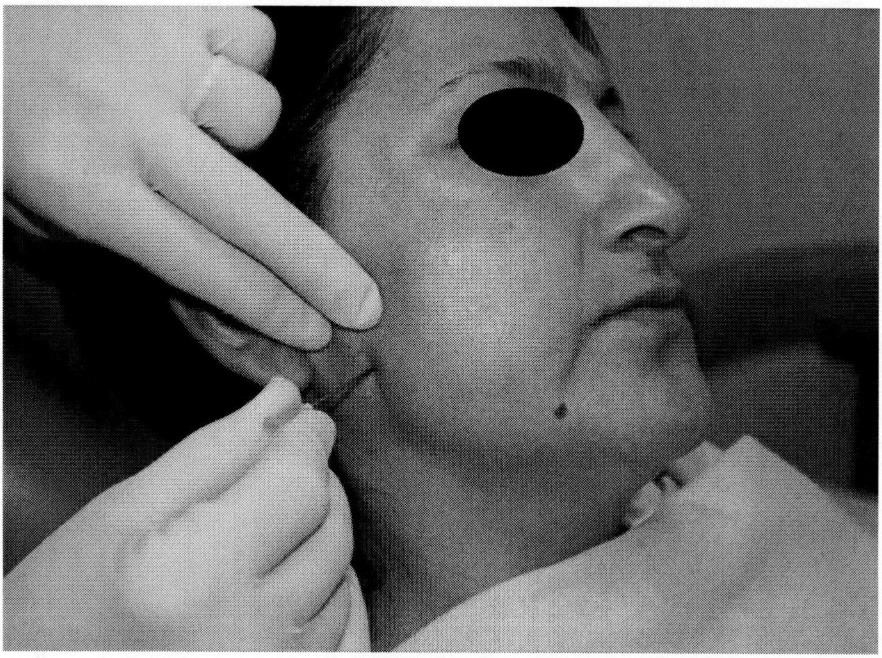

B. (Continued).

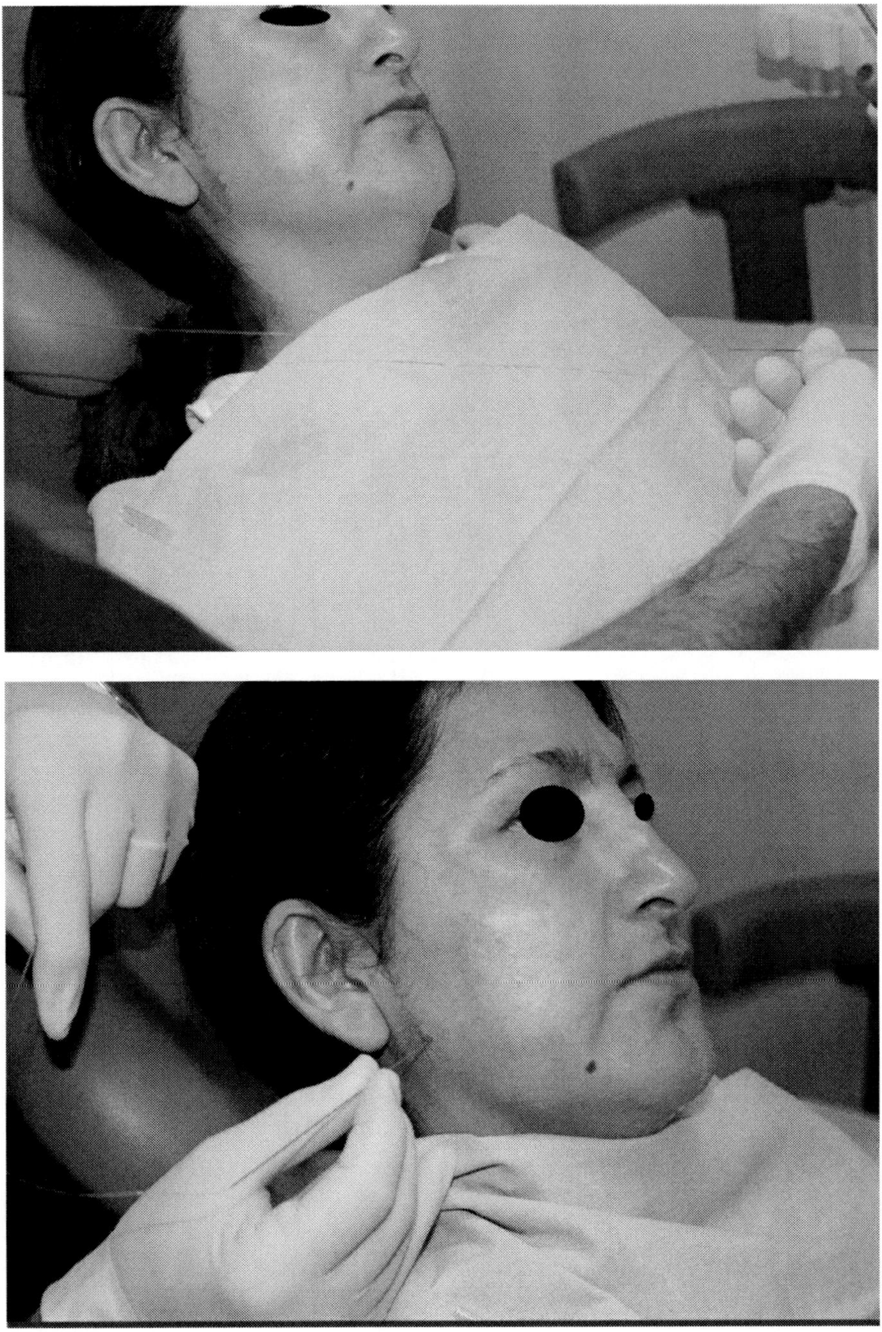

B. (Continued).

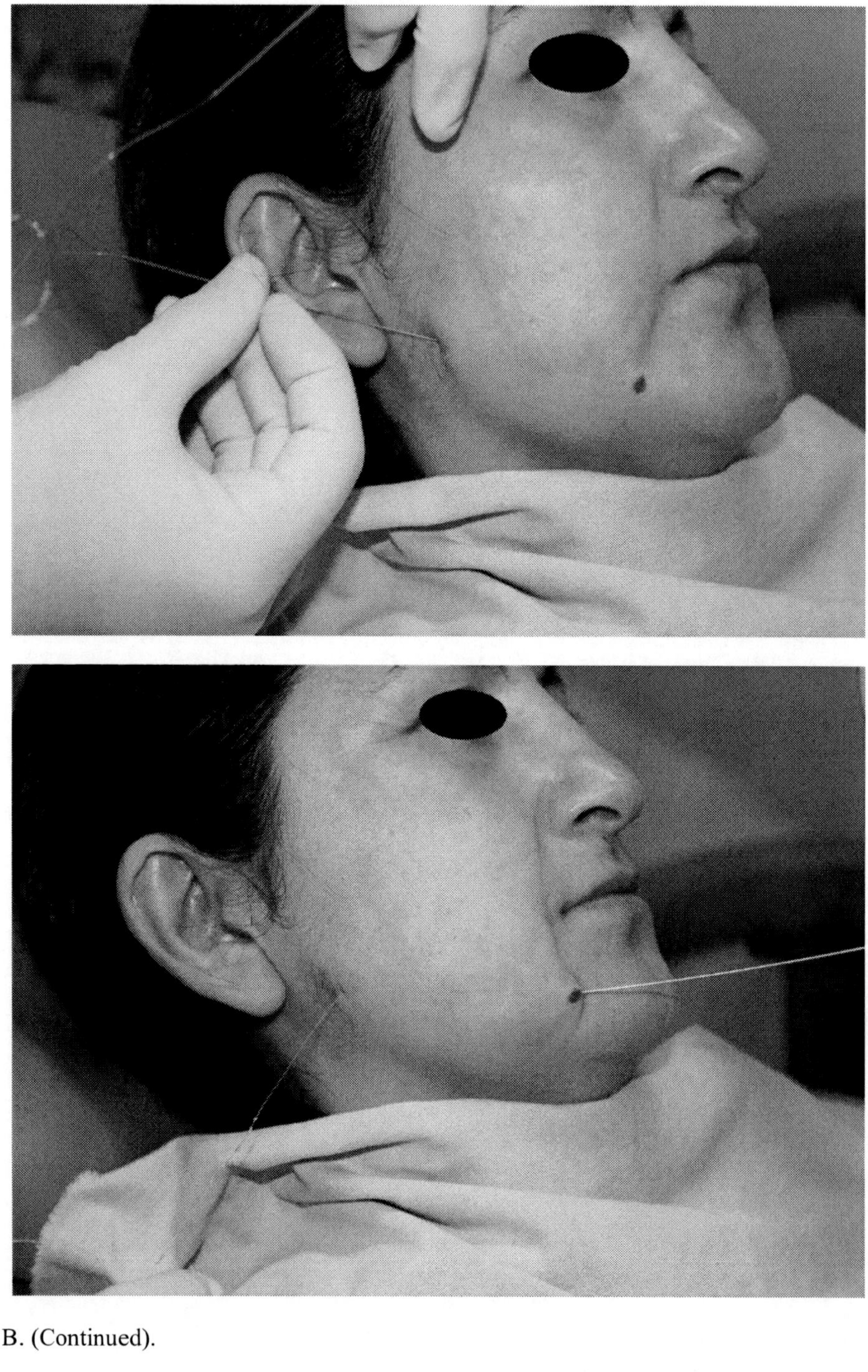

B. (Continued).

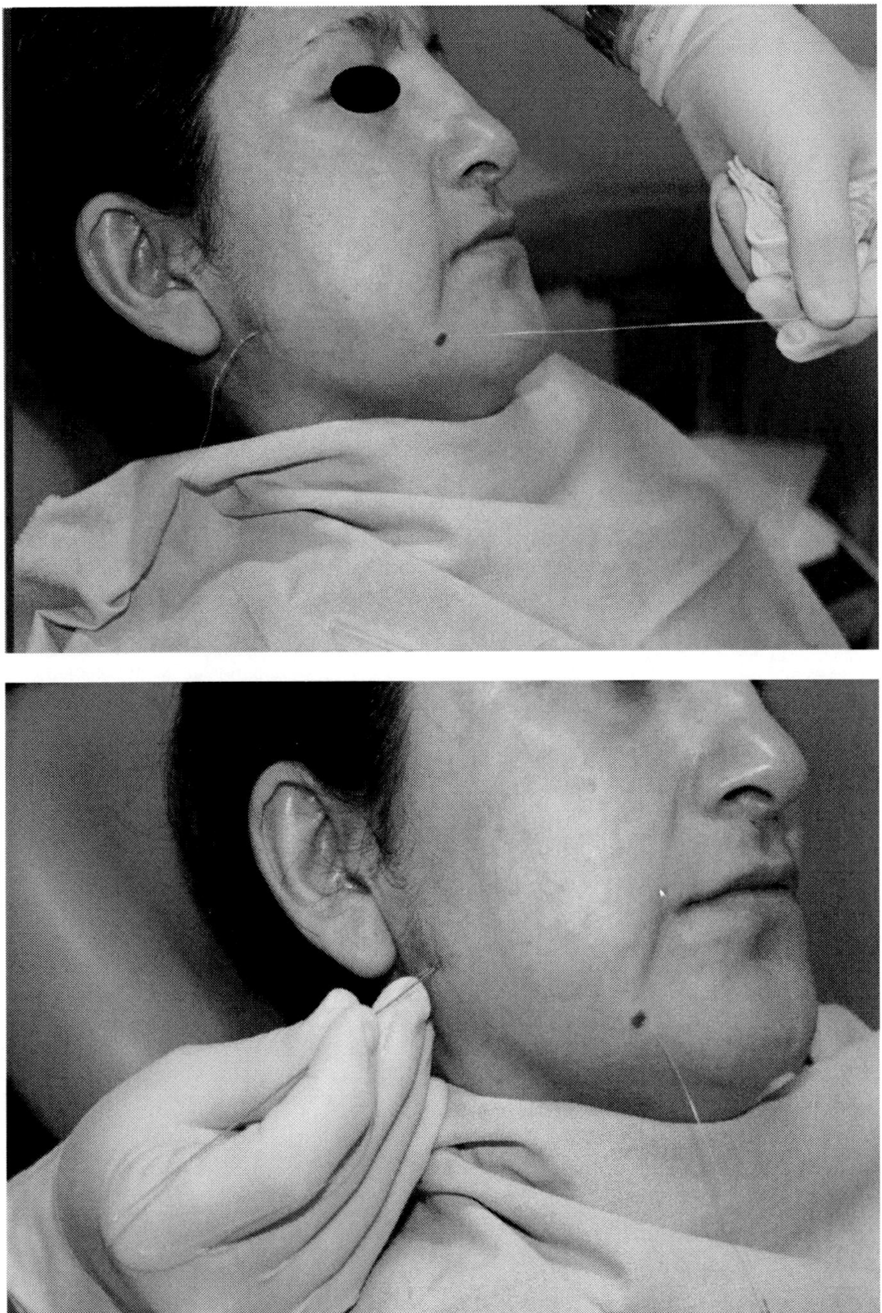

B. (Continued).

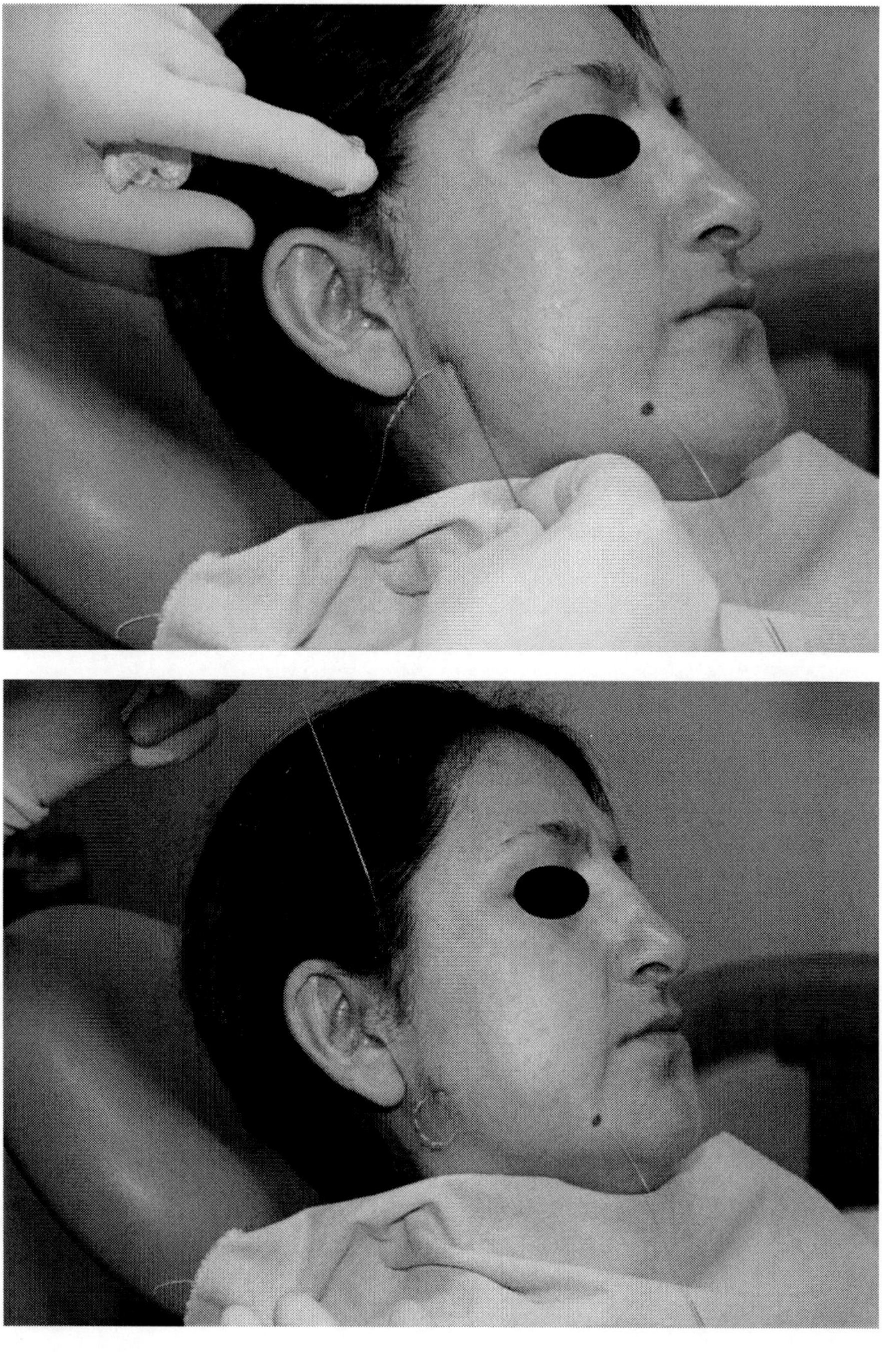

B. (Continued).

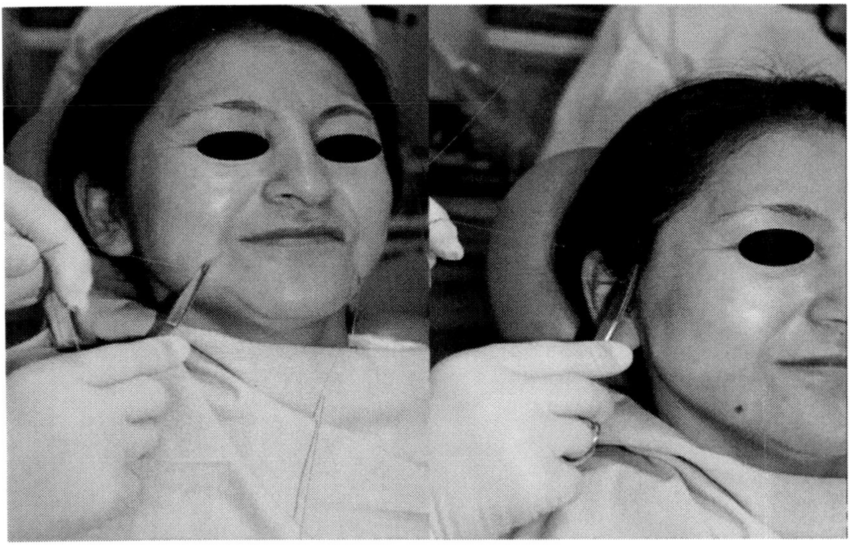

B: L shaped application of coned wire to lift the cheek: project (1); insertion of perforating needle (2); appropriate pre-surgical wire stripping (3); insertion of the guide needle (4); the needle is directed to the desired target point (5); complete insertion of the first half of the coned wire (6); wire stripping is used to be sure that all the cones are in the appropriate position (7); insertion of the guide needle for the second half of the wire (8); the second guide needle is directed to the desired target point (9); appliance of the appropriate tension on the wire provides the subcutaneous entrance of the cones (10); after the application the portion of the wire remaining out of the skin is removed by scissors (11).

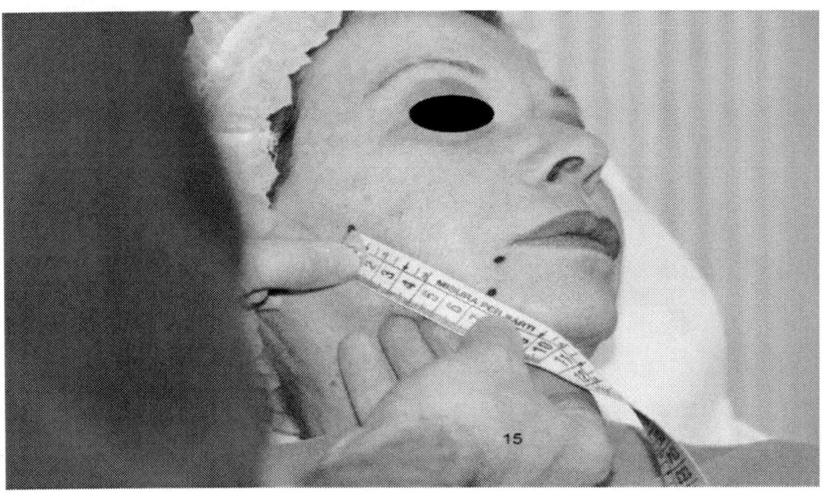

C. (Continued).

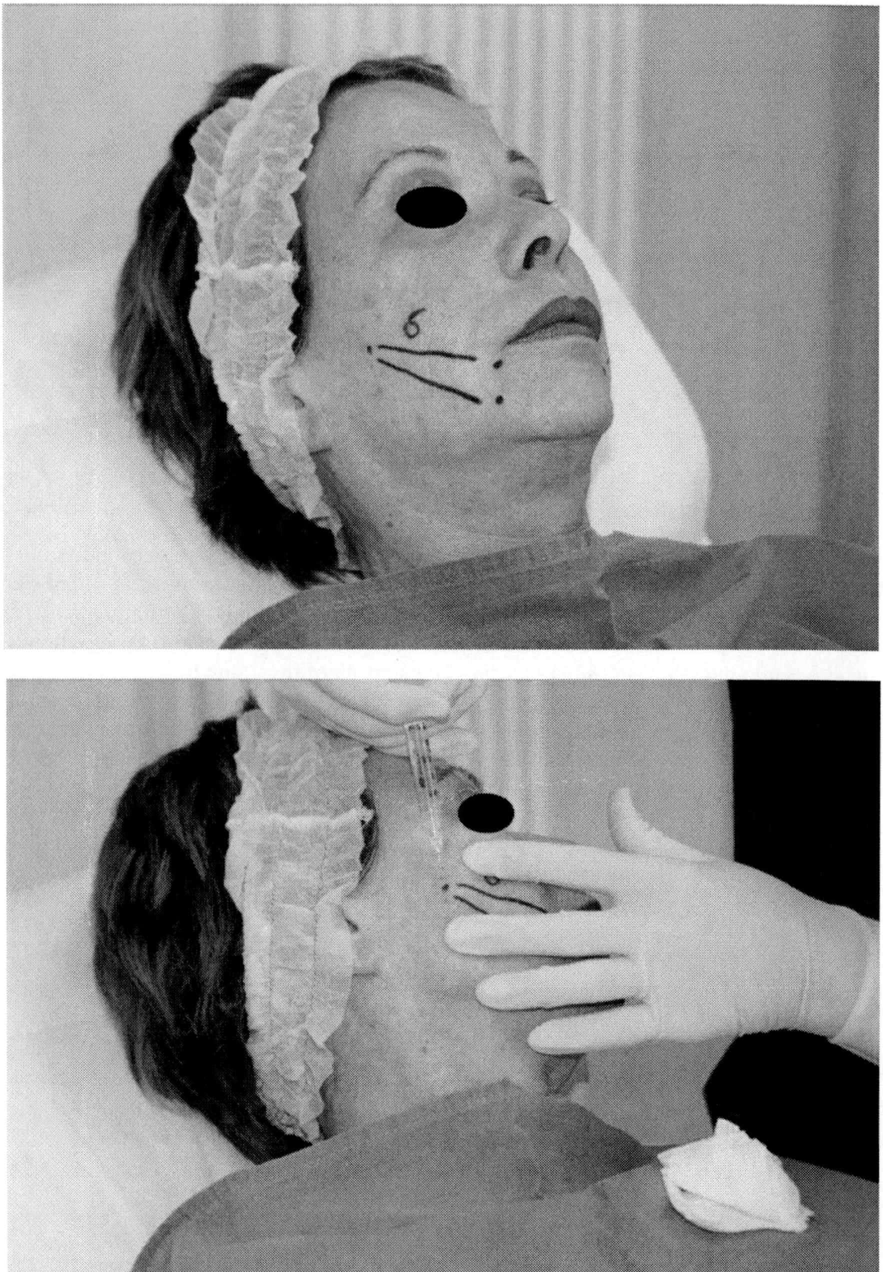

C. (Continued).

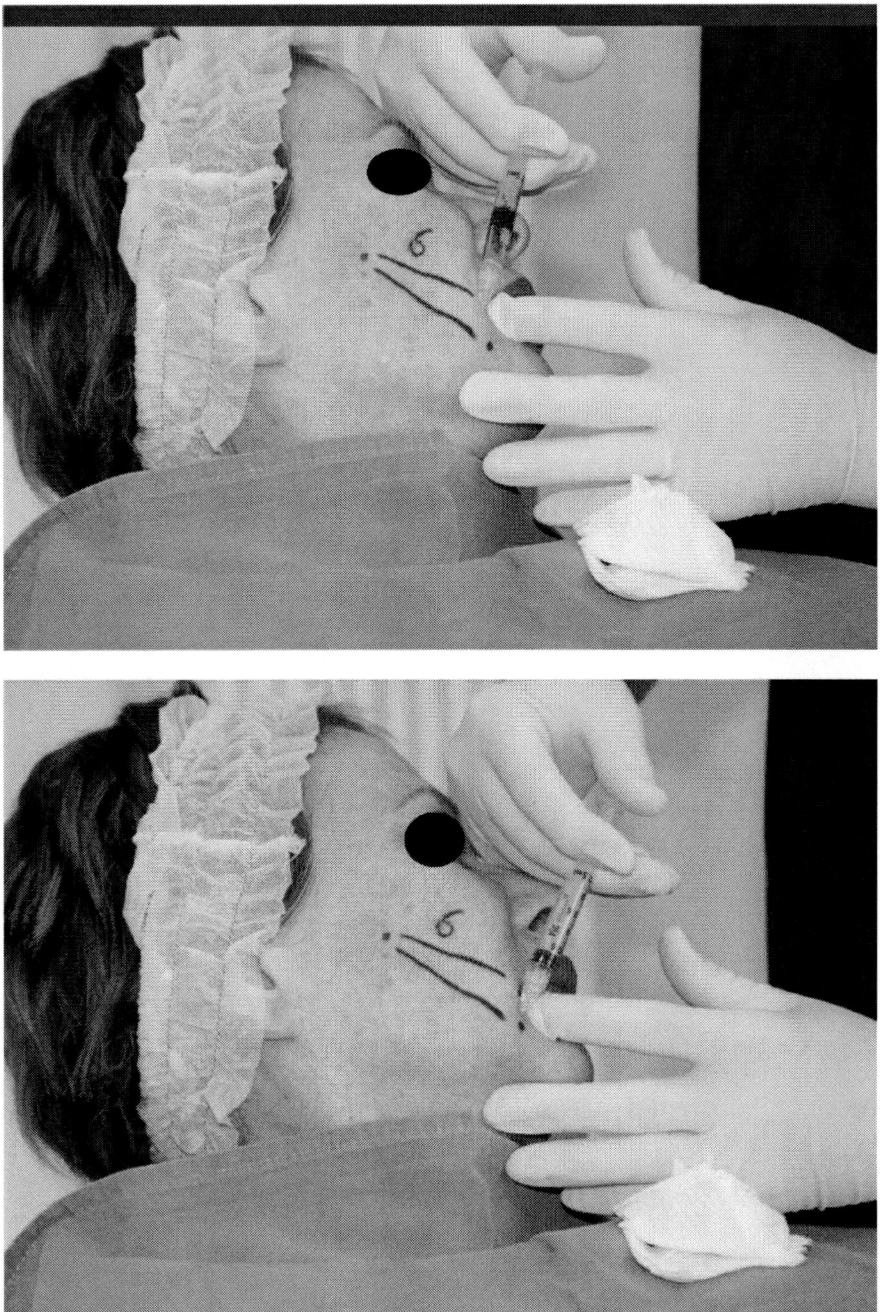

C. (Continued).

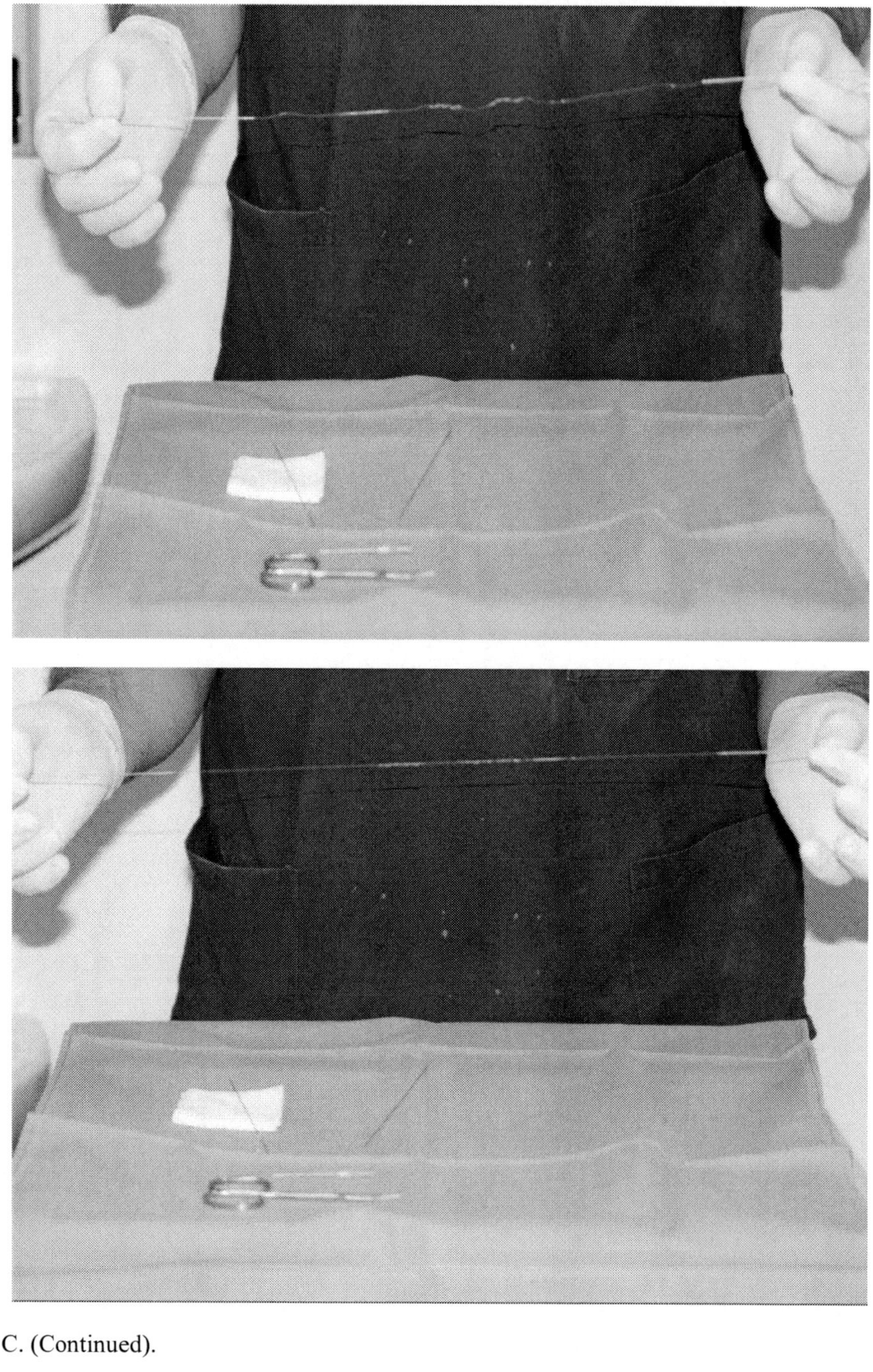

C. (Continued).

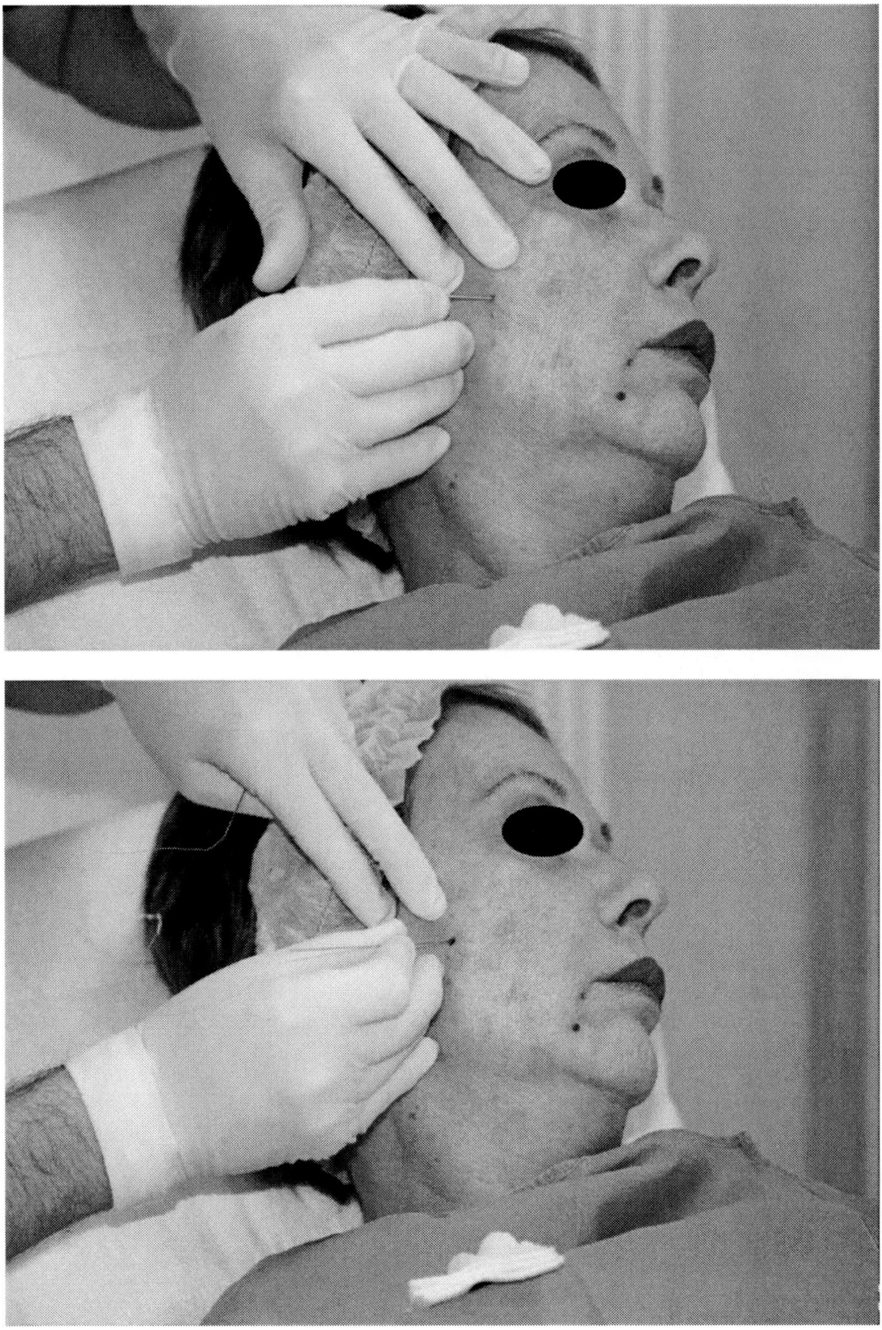

C. (Continued).

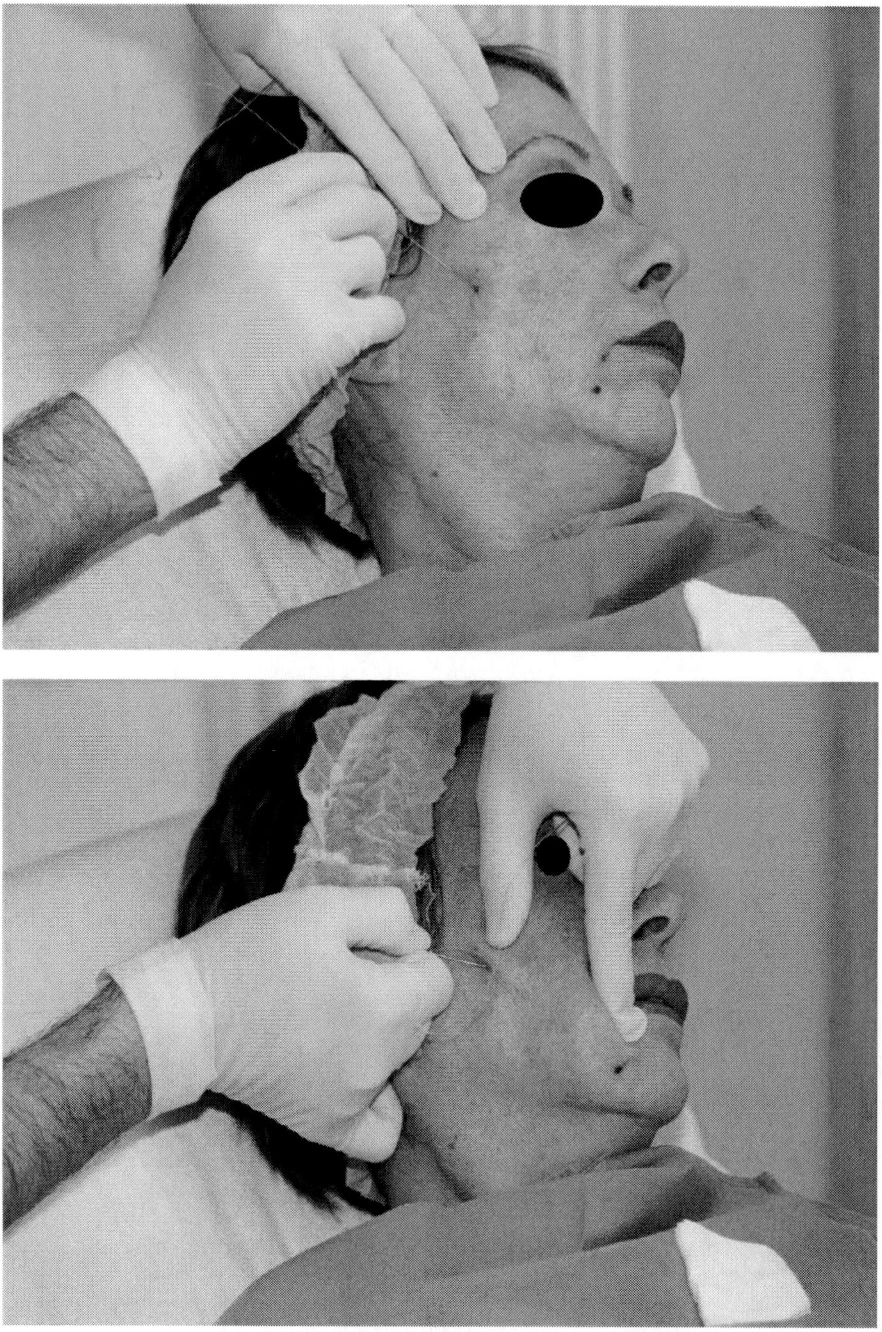

C. (Continued).

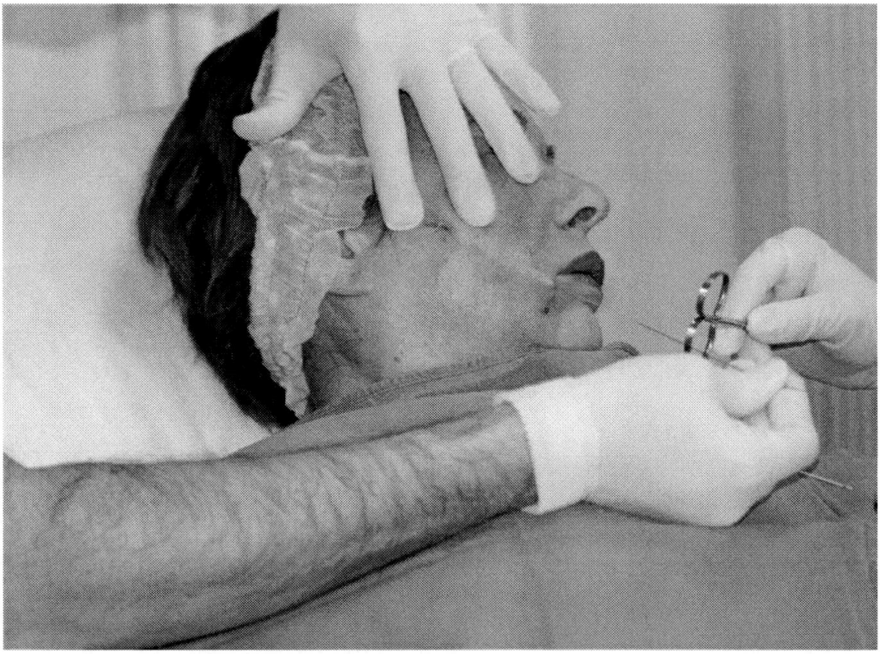

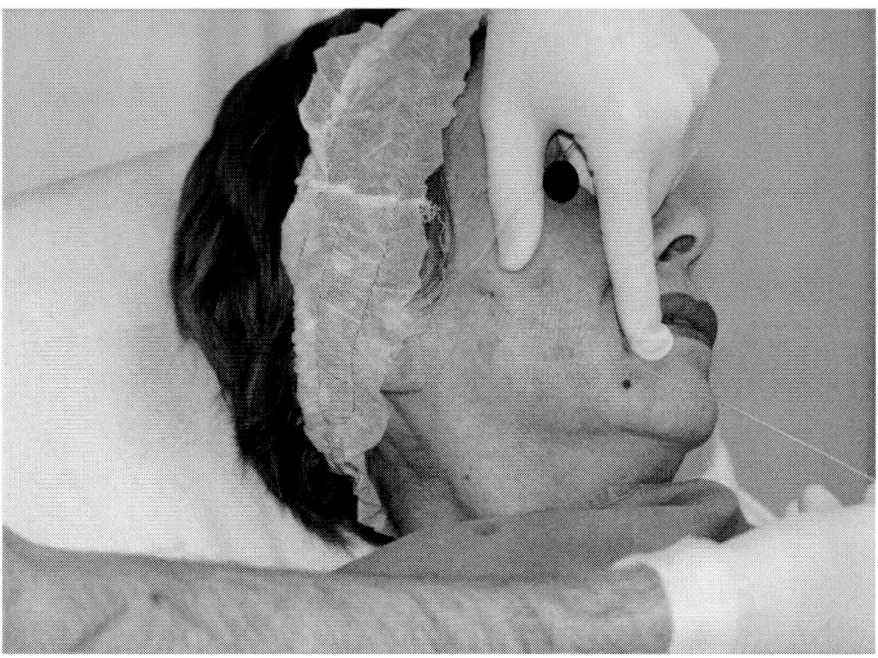

C. (Continued).

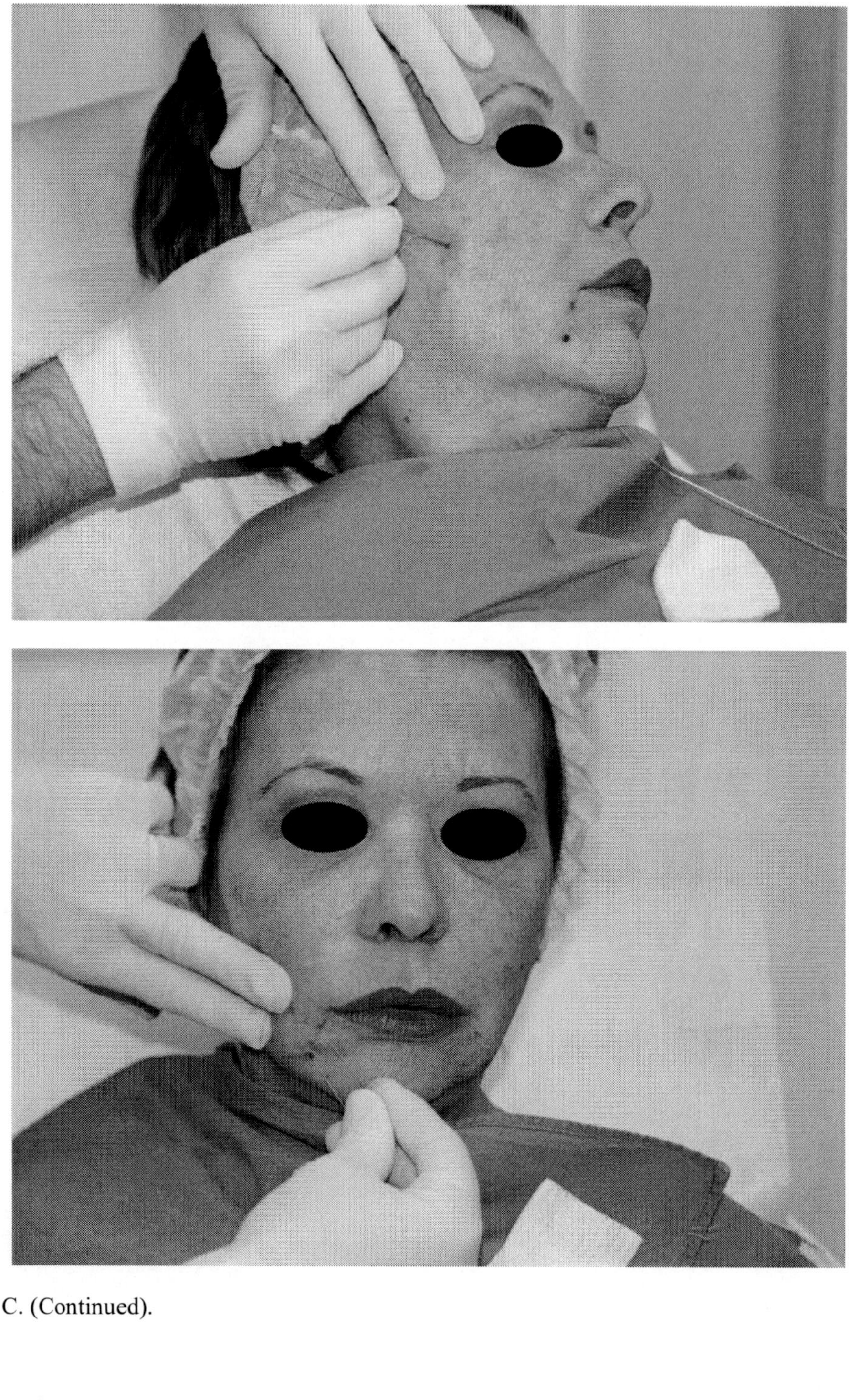

C. (Continued).

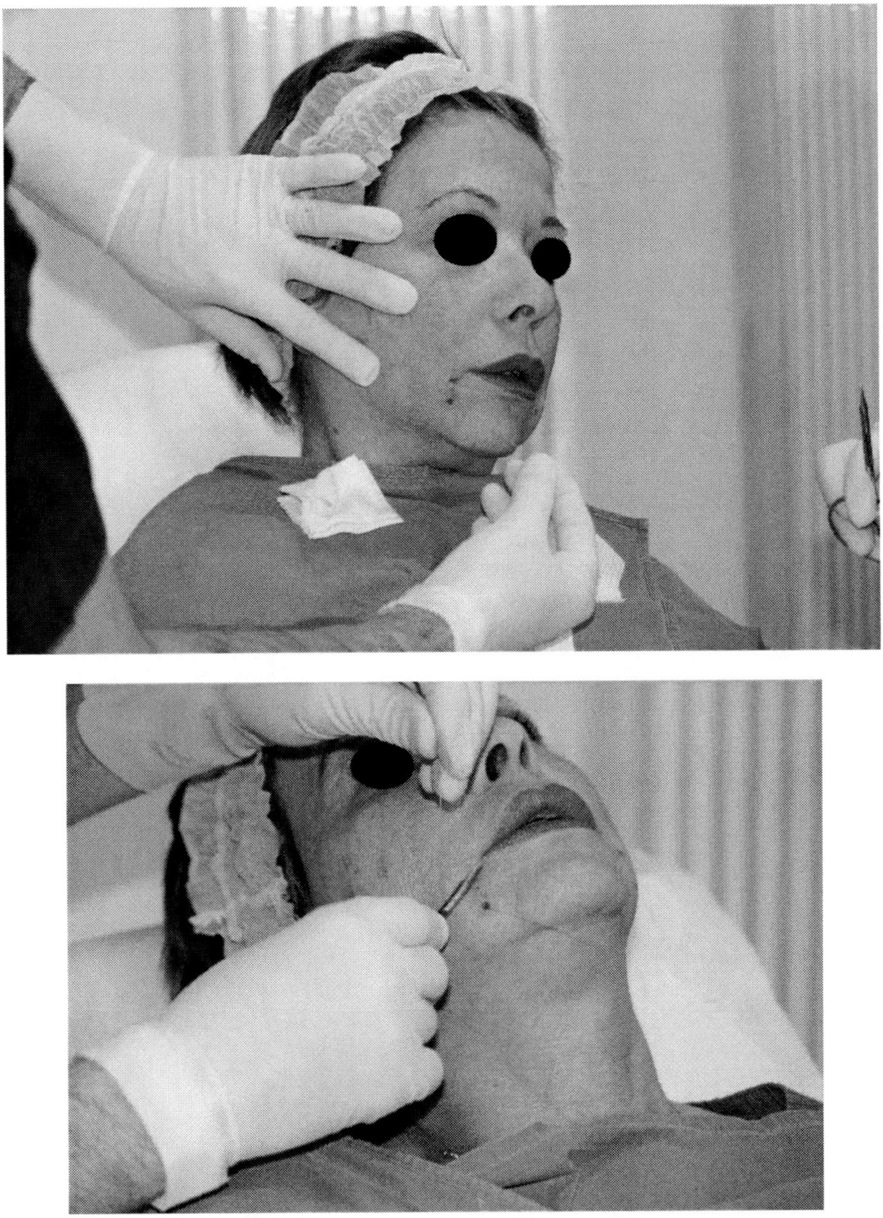

C. (Continued).

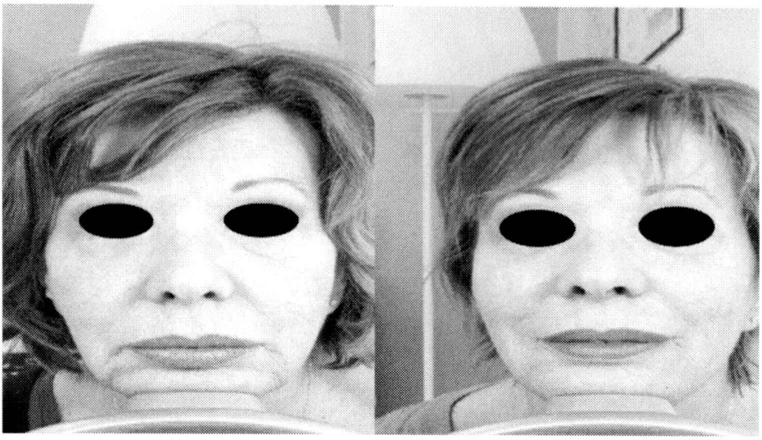

C: V shaped application of coned wire to lift the cheek: project (1,2); local anesthetic is injected on the cutaneous points in which the needle will enter (3) and exit (4,5) the skin; appropriate stripping of the wire (6,7) is needed before application; insertion of perforating 18 g needle (8); insertion of the guide needle of the first half of the wire (9); the needle is directed to the desired target point (10) and exits the skin (11,12); wire stripping is used to be sure that all the cones are in the appropriate position (13); insertion of the guide needle for the second half of the wire (14); once the two halves of the wire are inserted, appropriate tension (15) will lead to tissue remodeling (16); after the application the portion of the wire remaining out of the skin is removed by scissors (17); frontal pre and postsurgical photos (18).

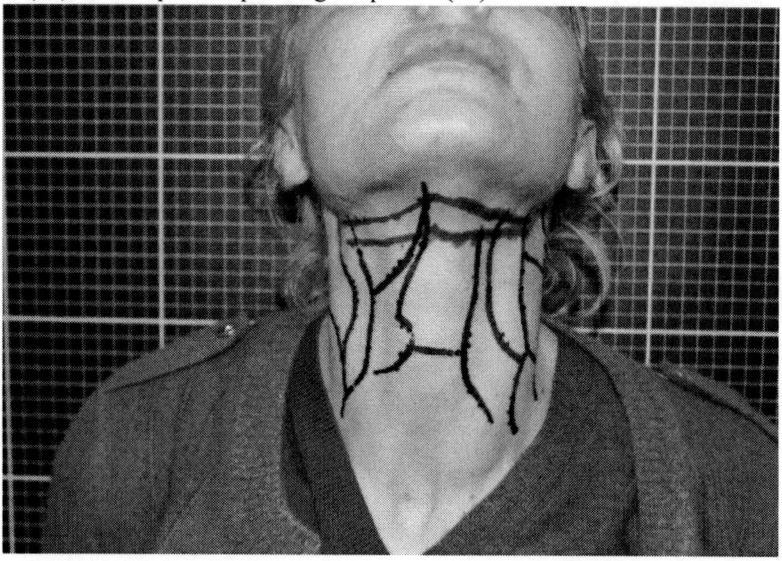

D. (Continued).

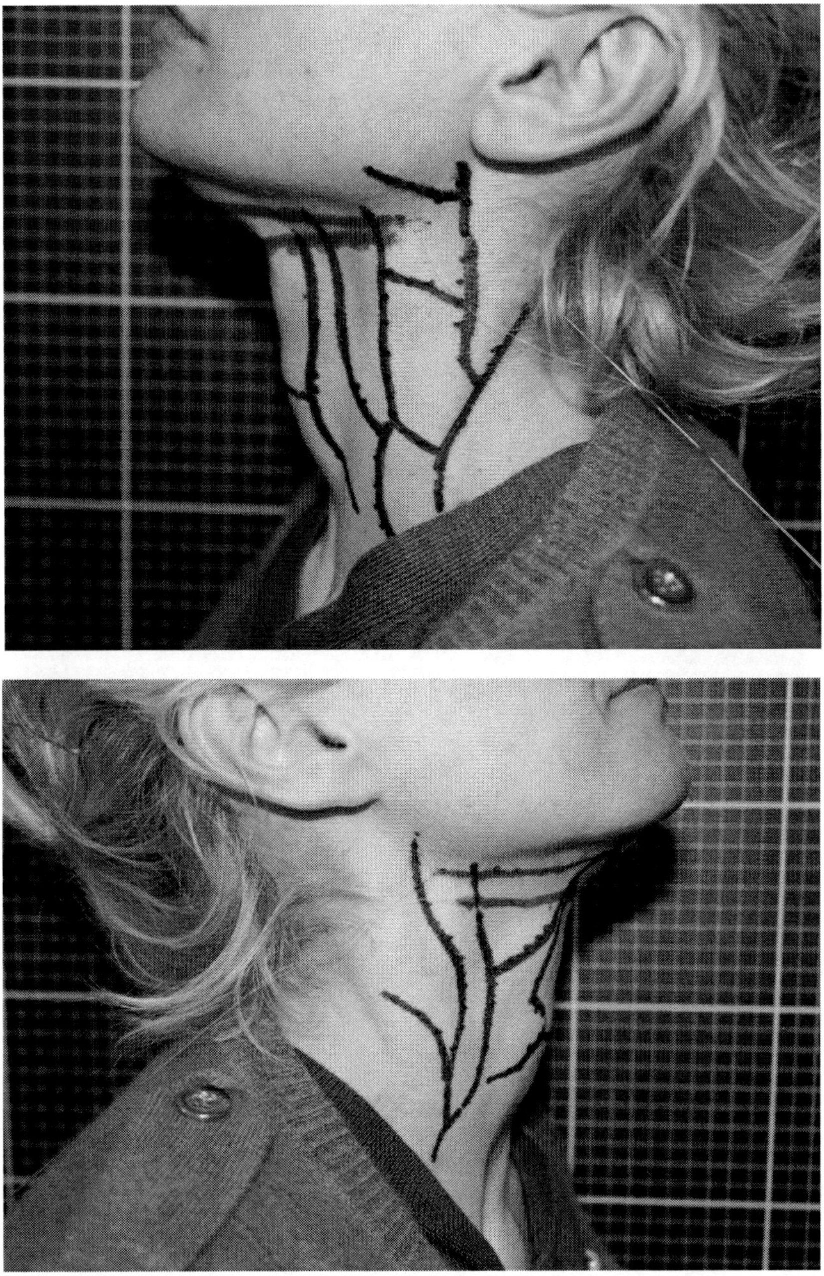

D: Topographical relationships between cervical applied coned wires and superficial vessels in cervical region on the frontal (1) and lateral (2,3) planes.

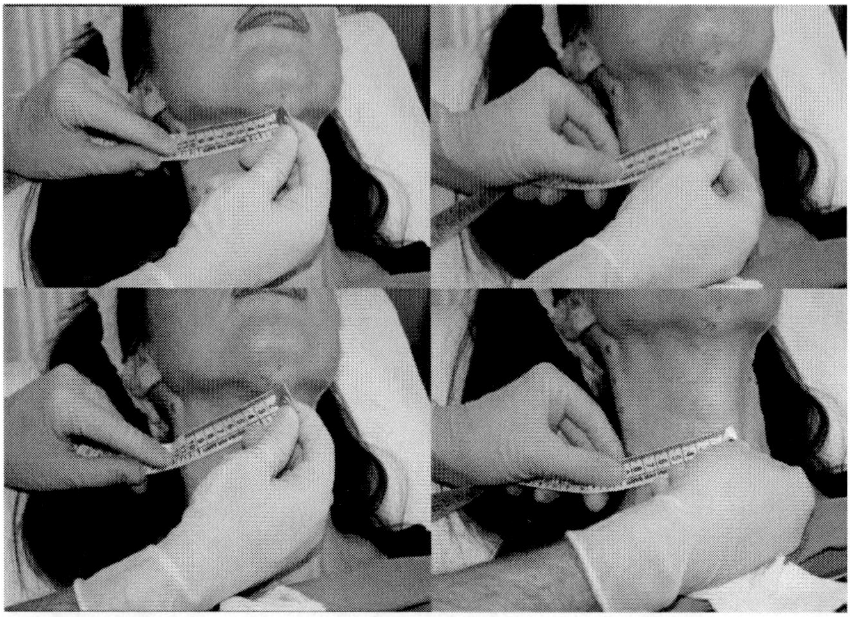

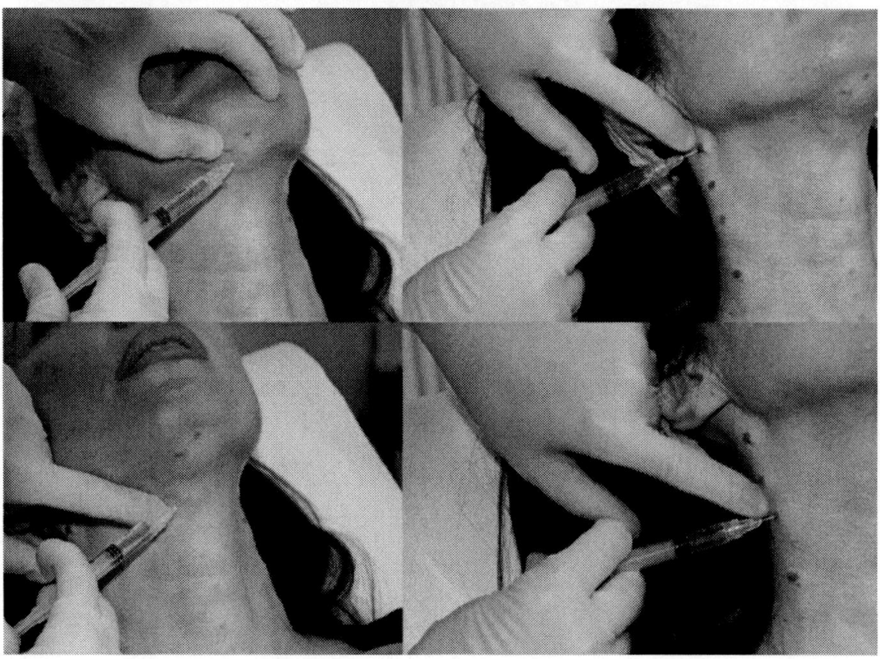

E. (Continued).

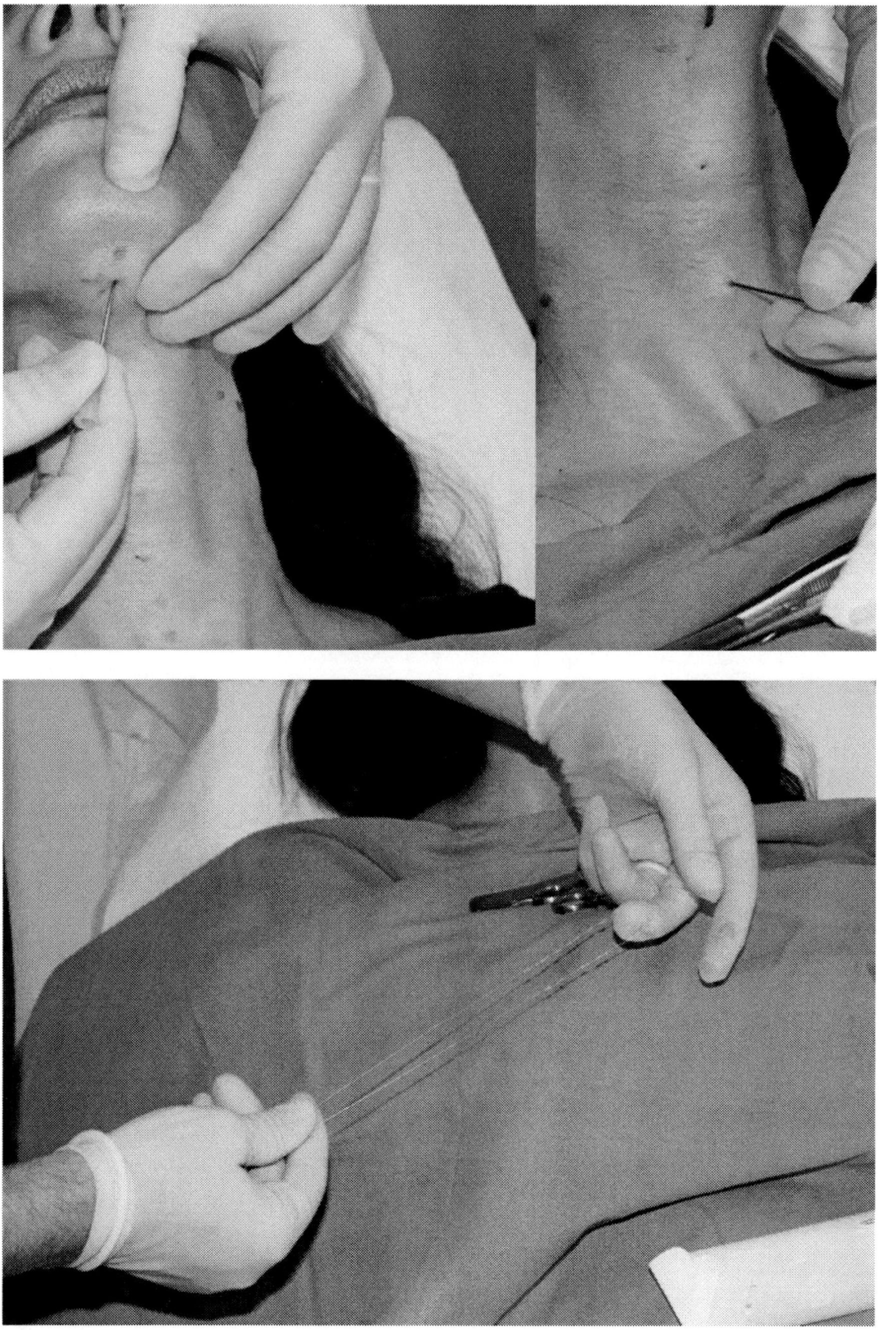

E. (Continued).

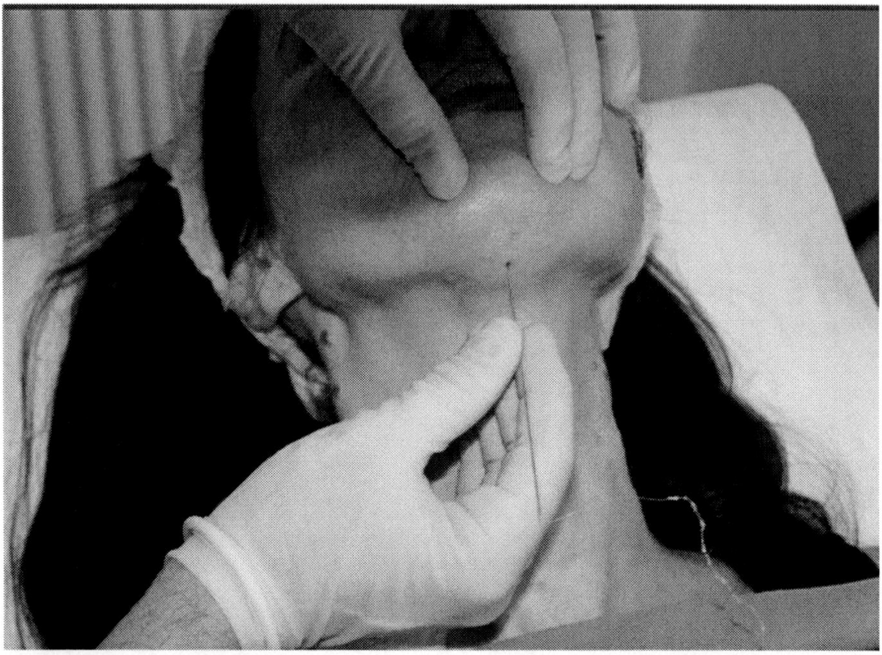

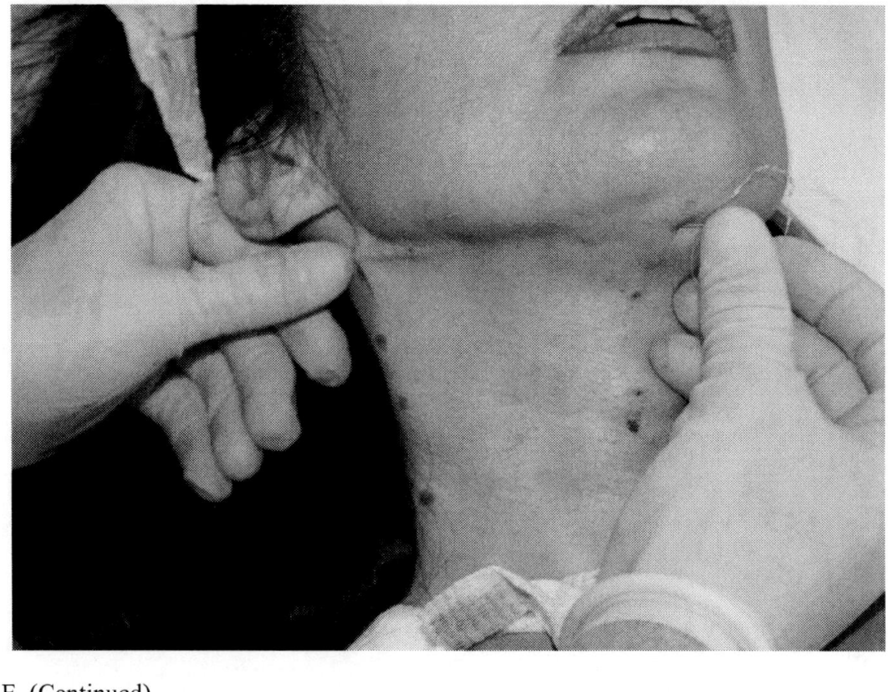

E. (Continued).

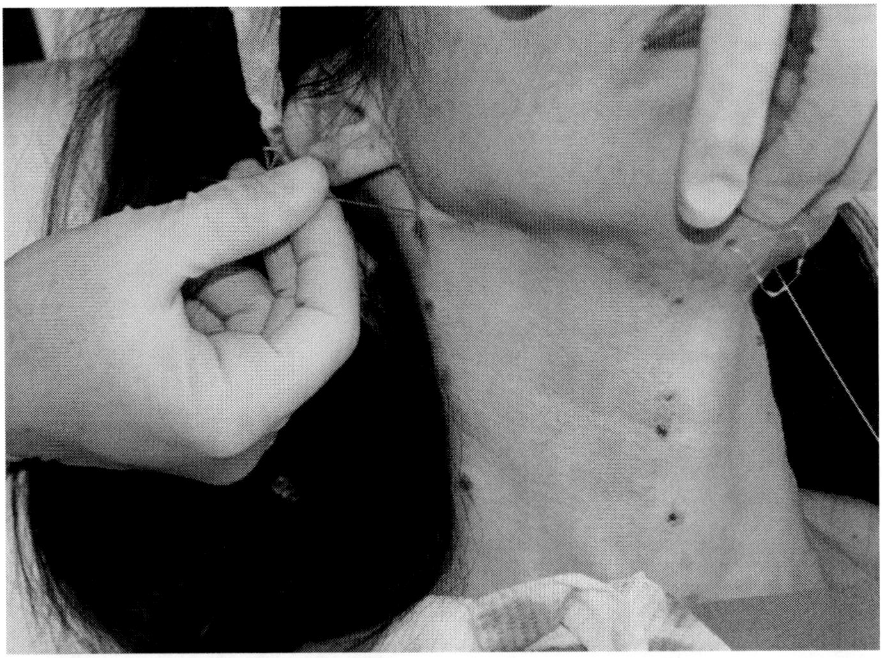

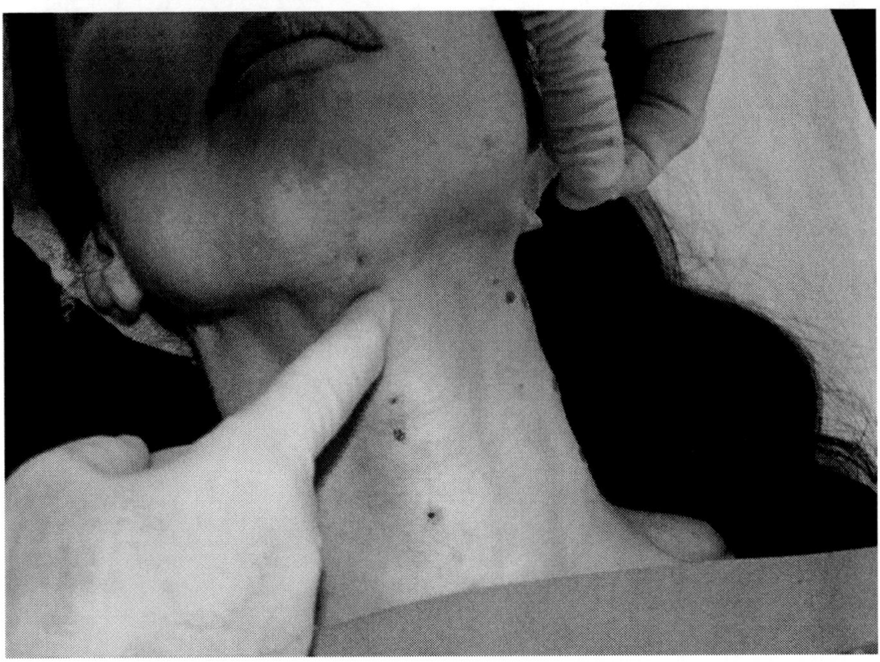

E. (Continued).

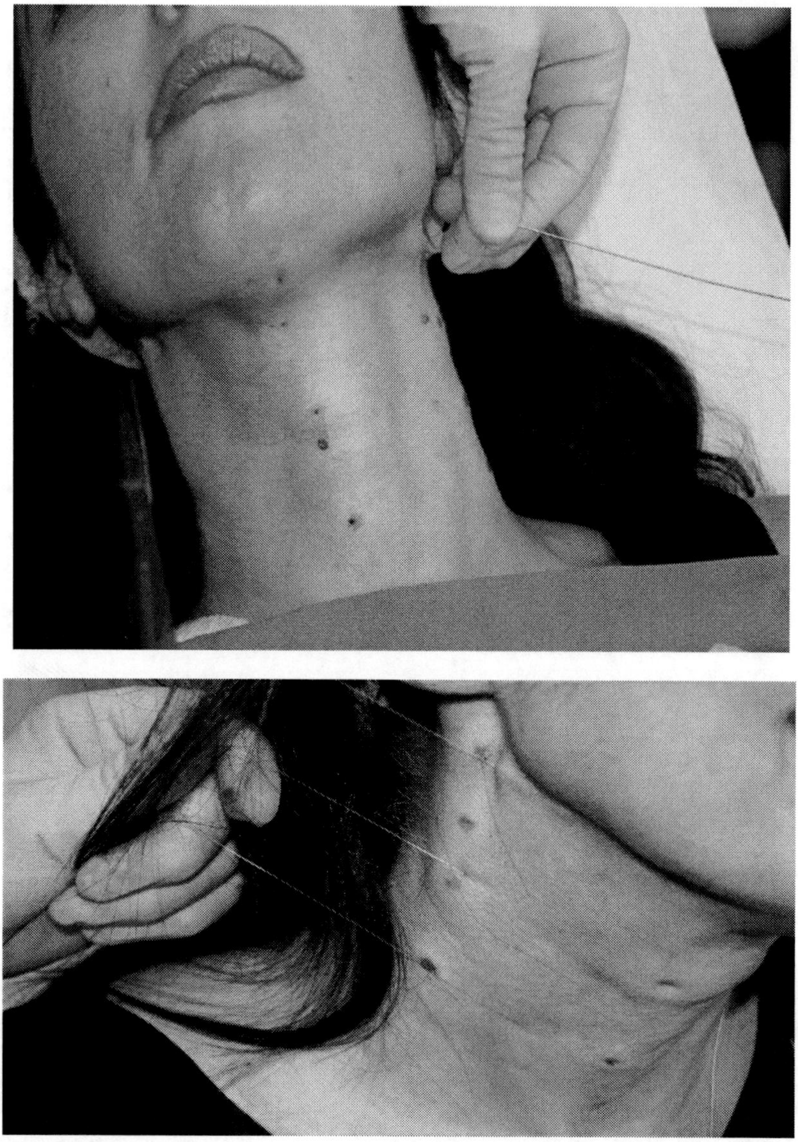

E. (Continued).

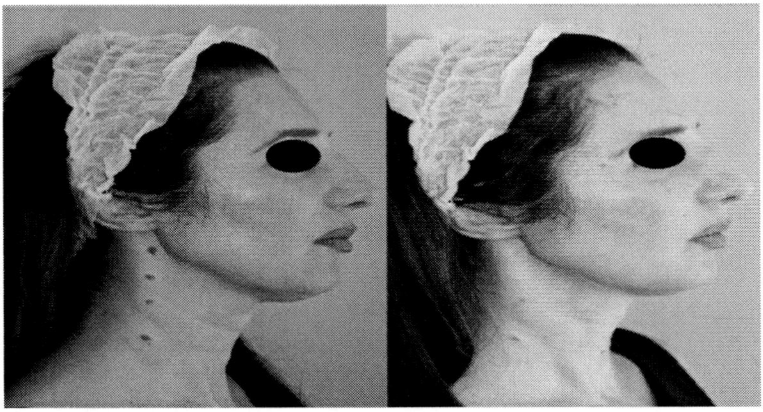

E: Multiple coned wires application to lift the cervical region: project (1); injection of local anesthetic (2); insertion of skin perforating 18 g needle (3) on the midline; appropriate stripping of the wire (4) is needed before application; insertion of the guide needle of the first half of the wire (5) on the midline; for cervical applications the guide needles of the two halves of the wired enter the skin on the midline and exit the cutaneous plane one for each side, allowing insertion of half of the wire on the right (6,7), and the other half on the left (8,9); this disposition is applied in order to provide optimal traction and maximize tissue repositioning (10); pre and postsurgical photos (11).

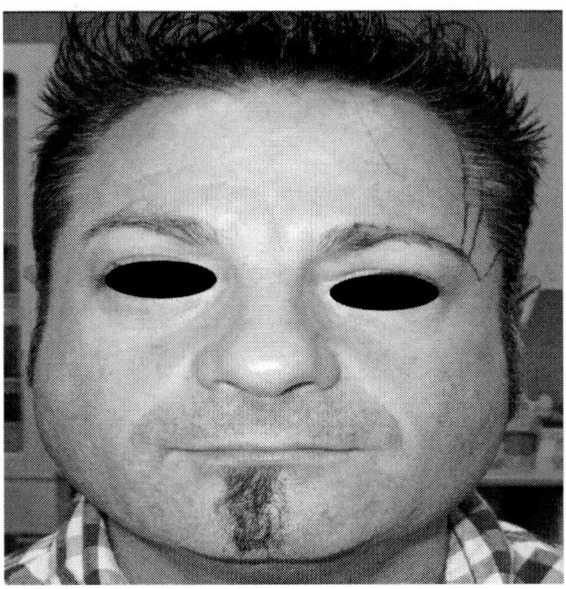

F. (Continued).

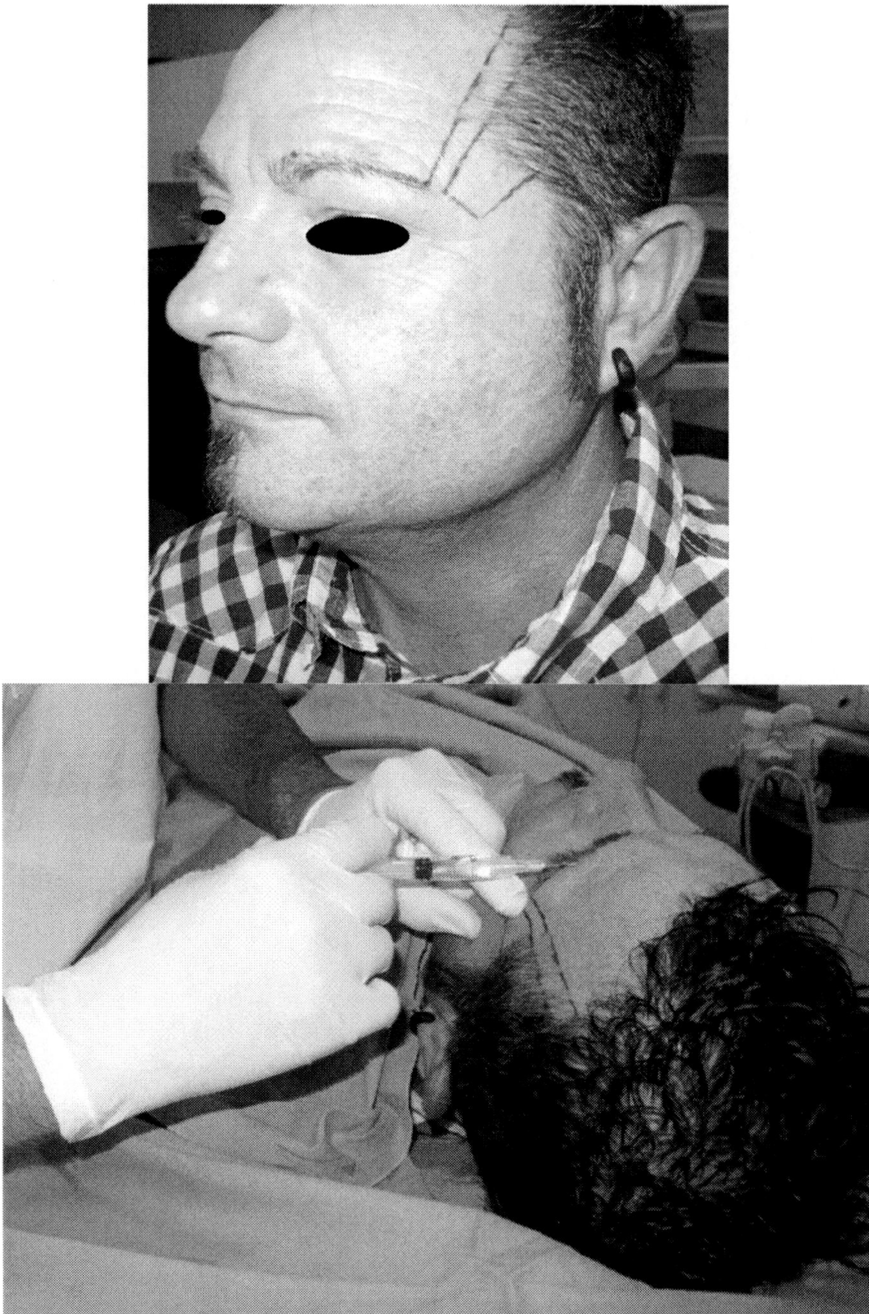

F. (Continued).

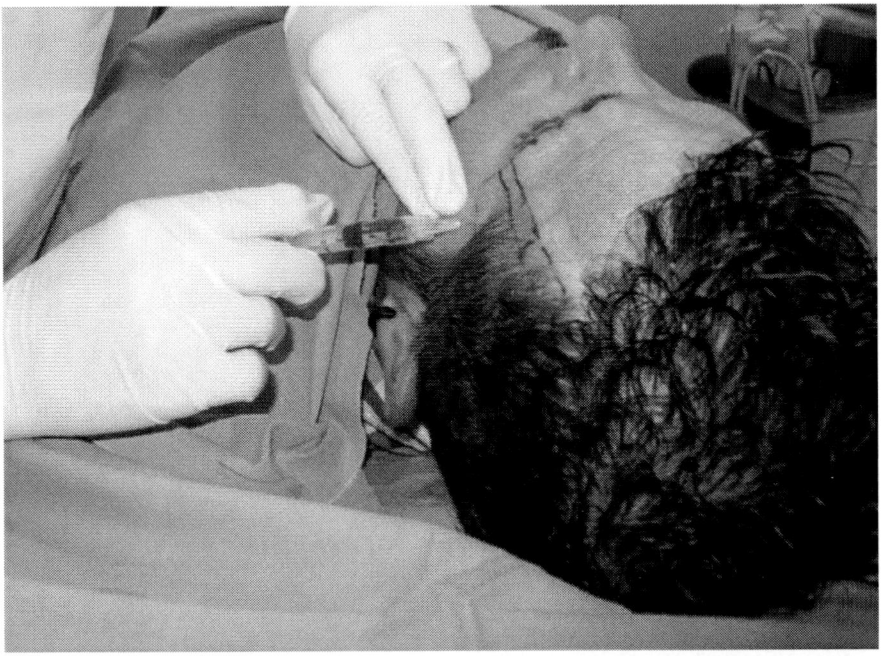

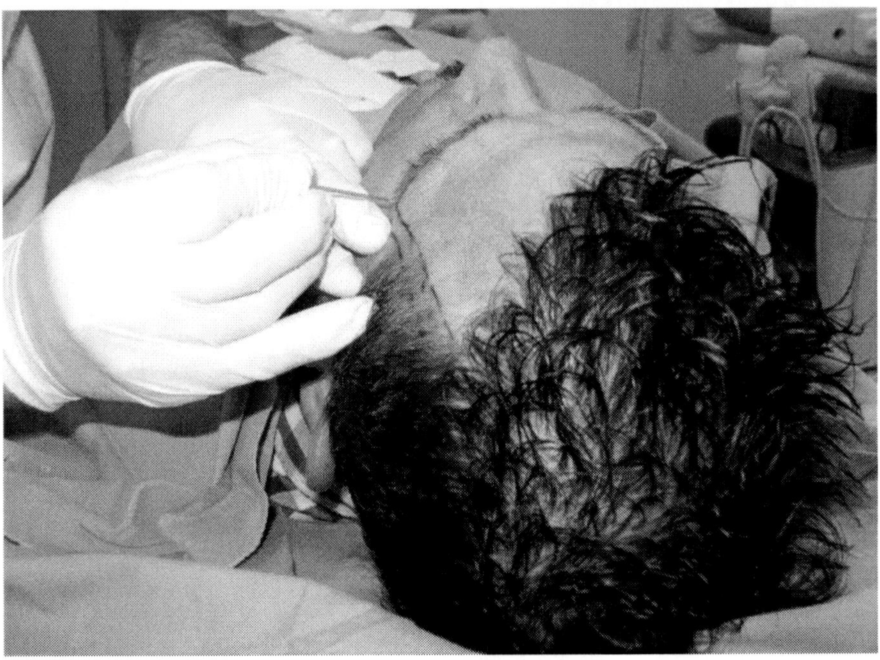

F. (Continued).

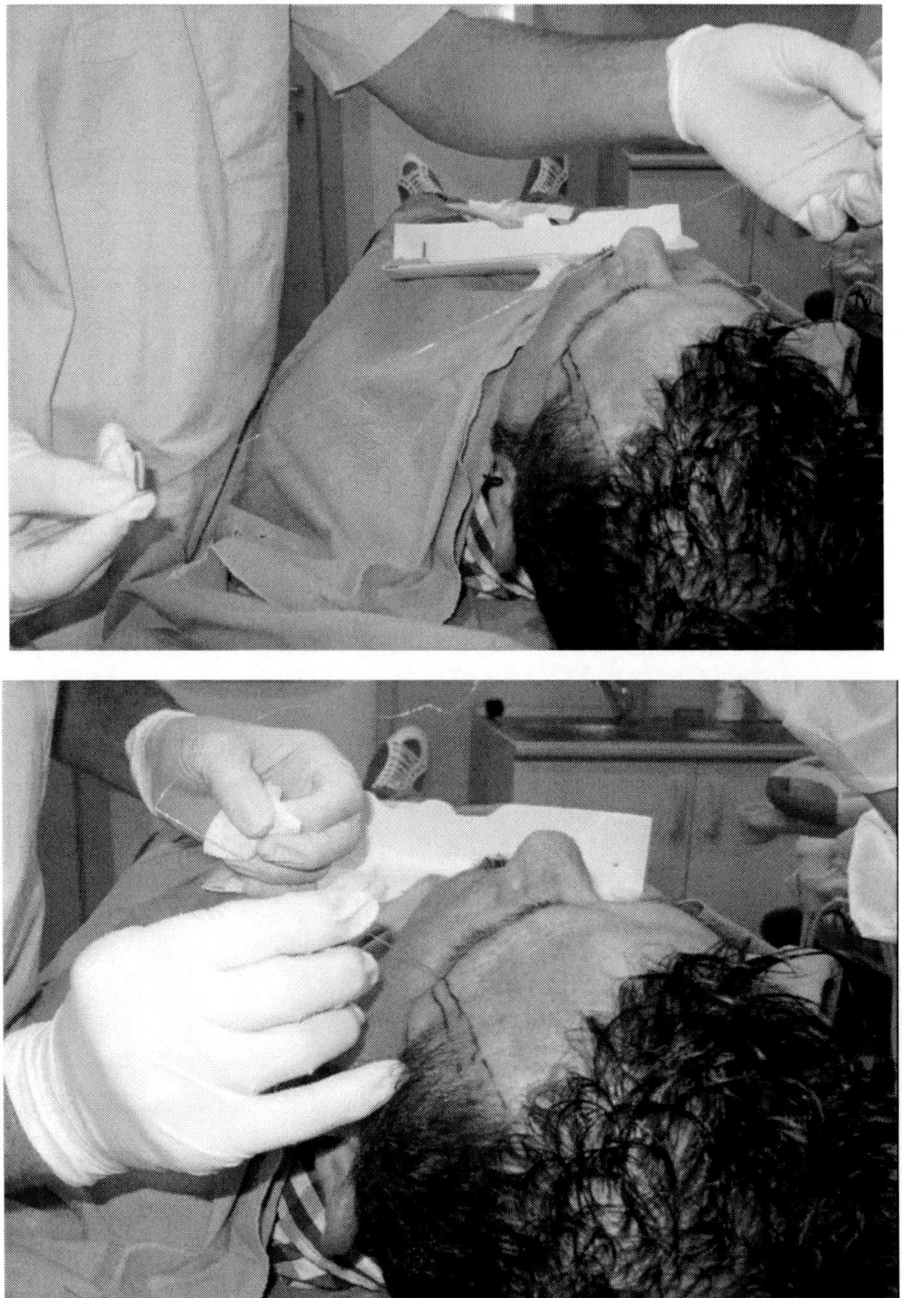

F. (Continued).

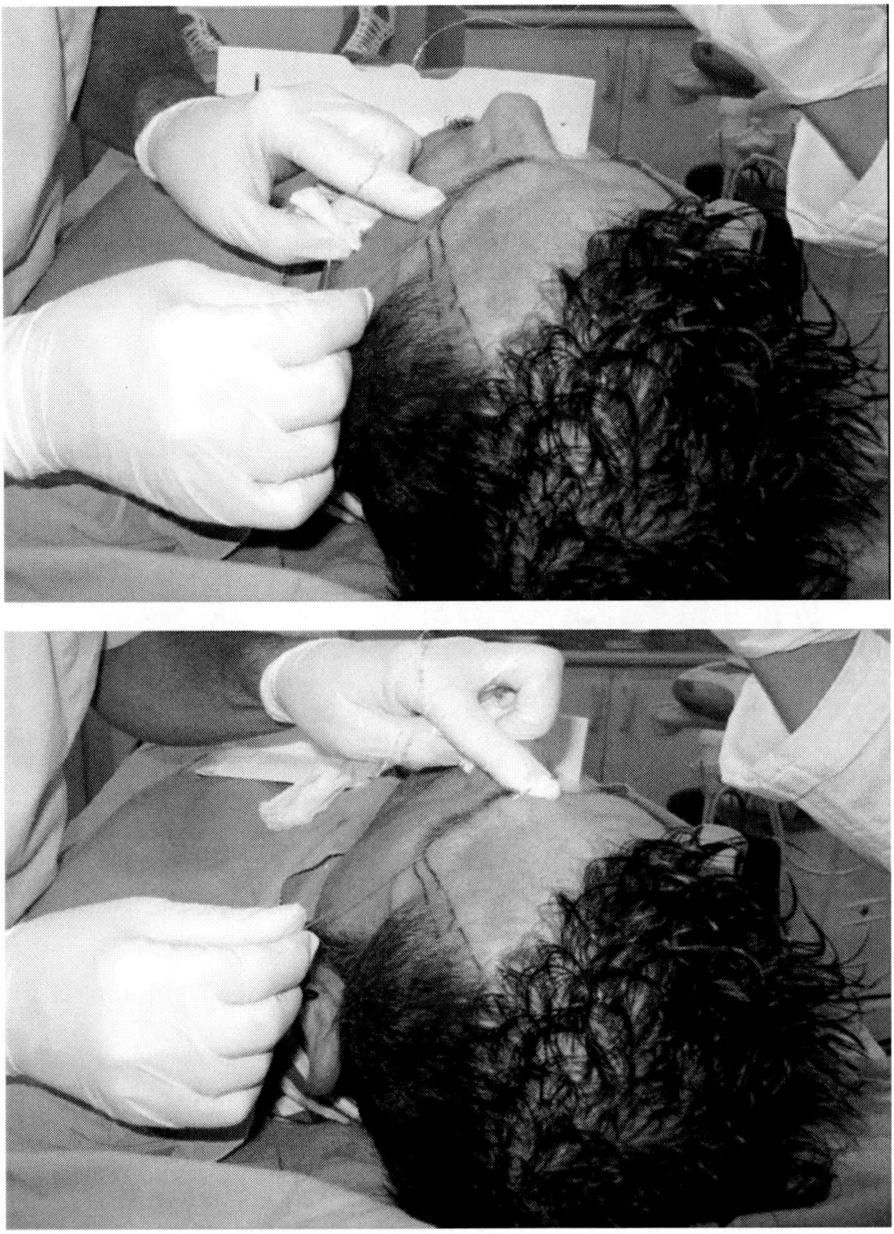

F. (Continued).

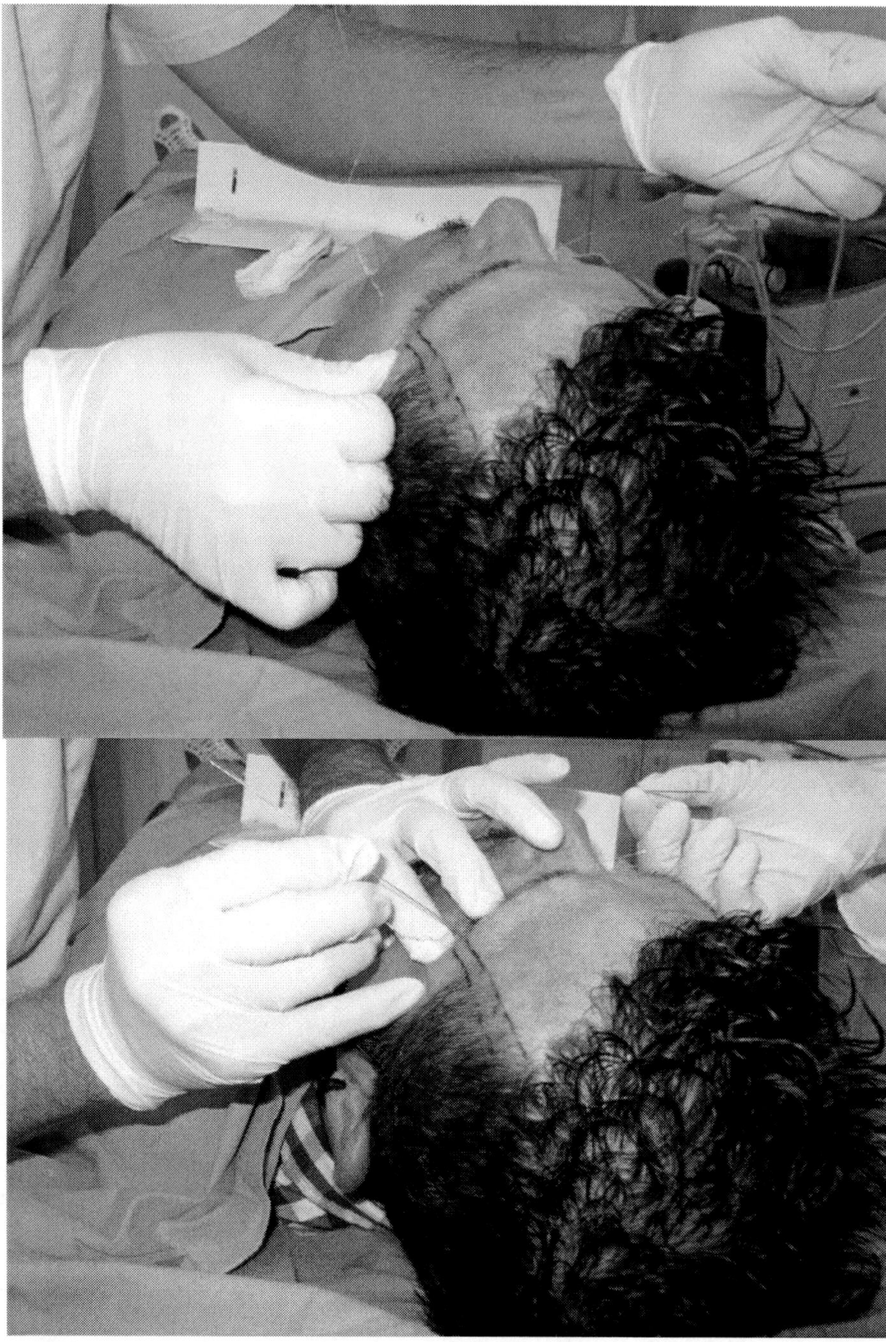

F. (Continued).

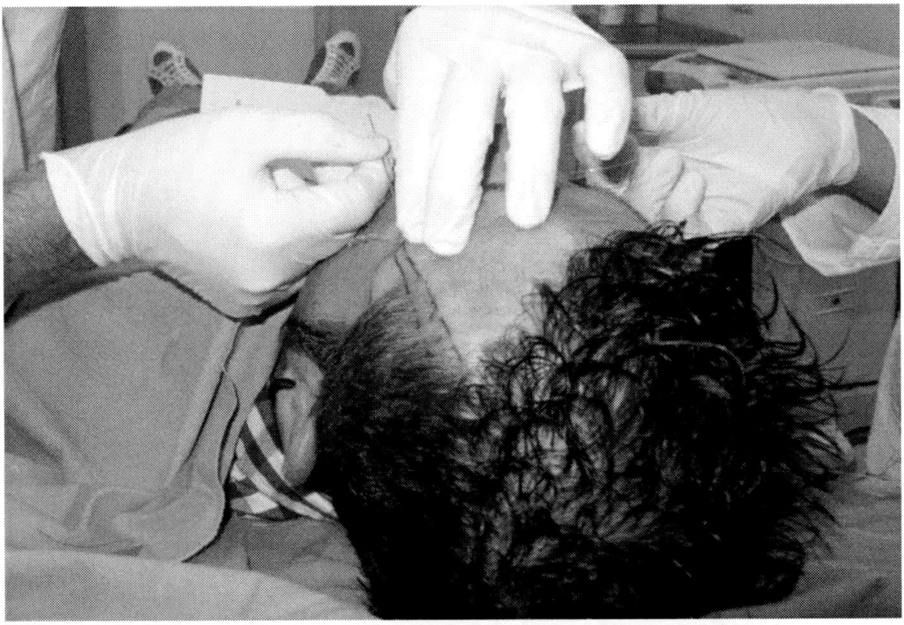

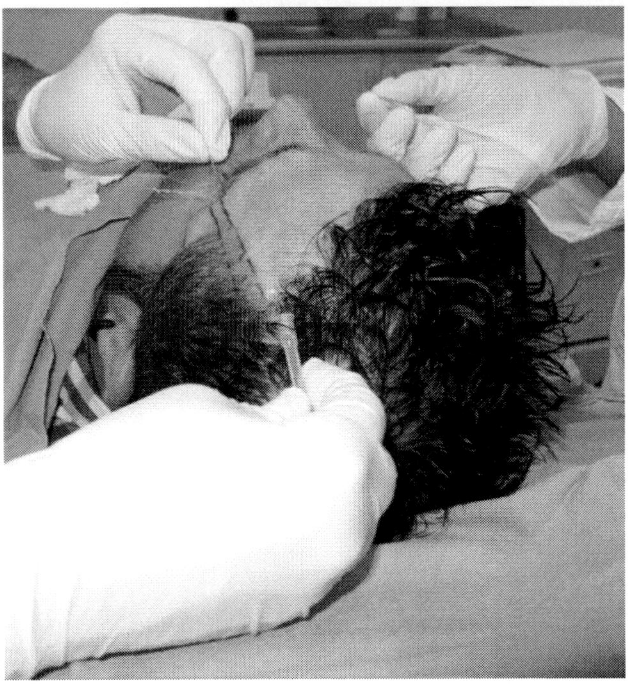

F. (Continued).

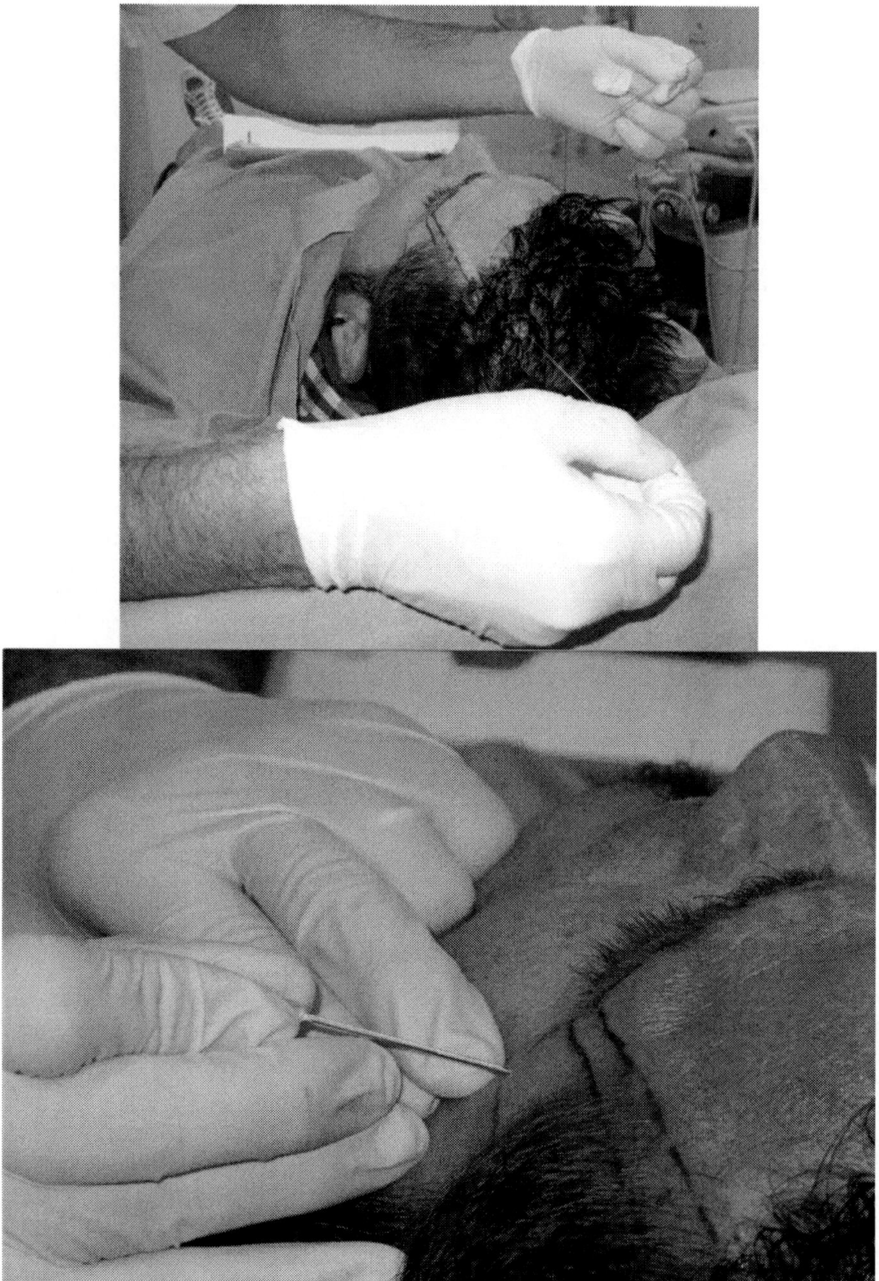

F. (Continued).

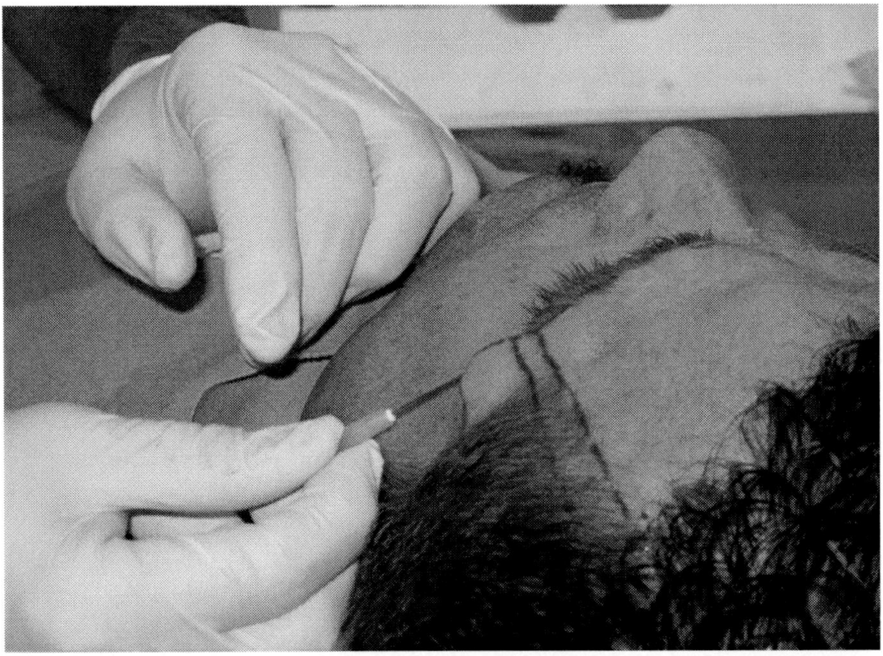

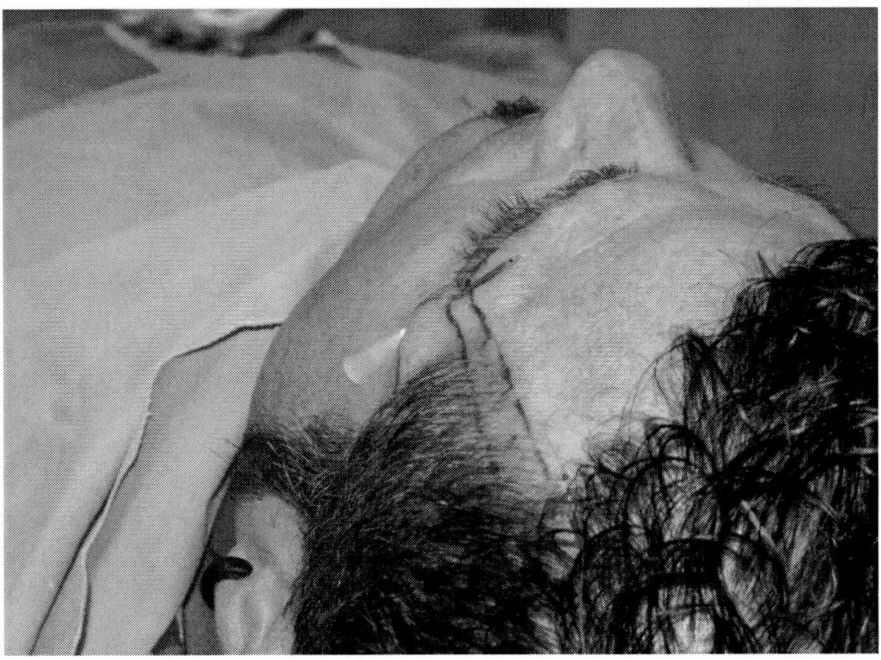

F. (Continued).

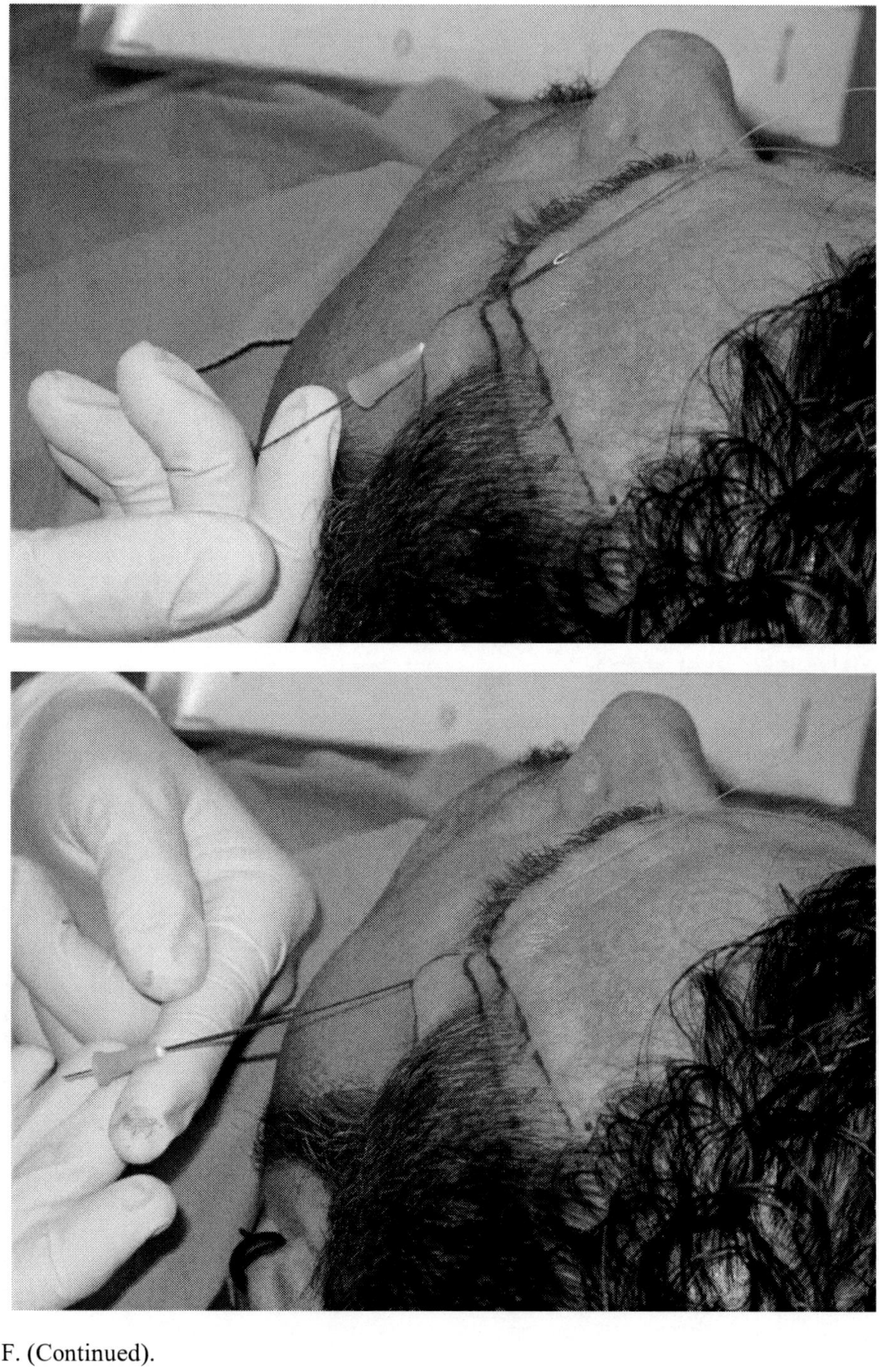

F. (Continued).

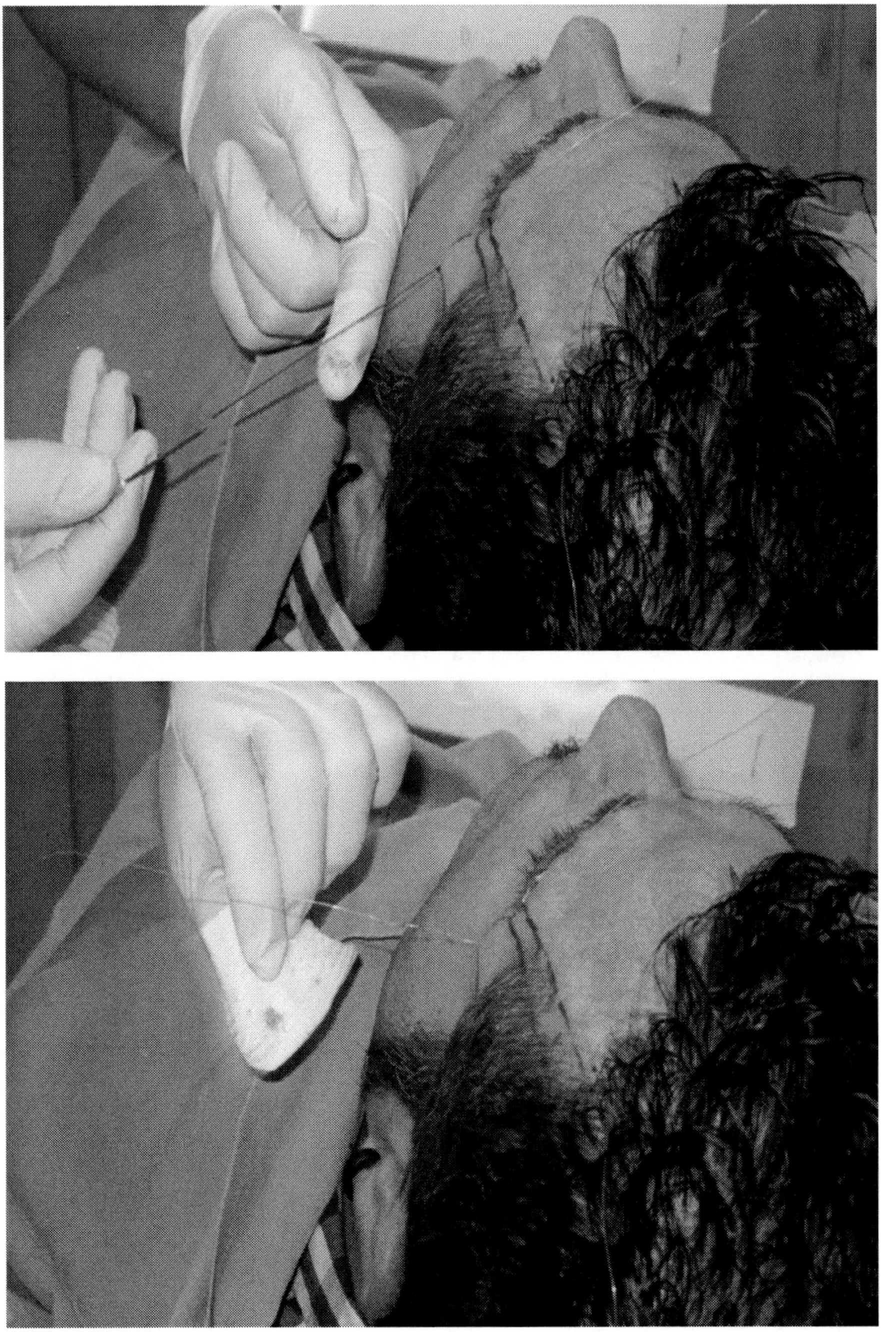

F. (Continued).

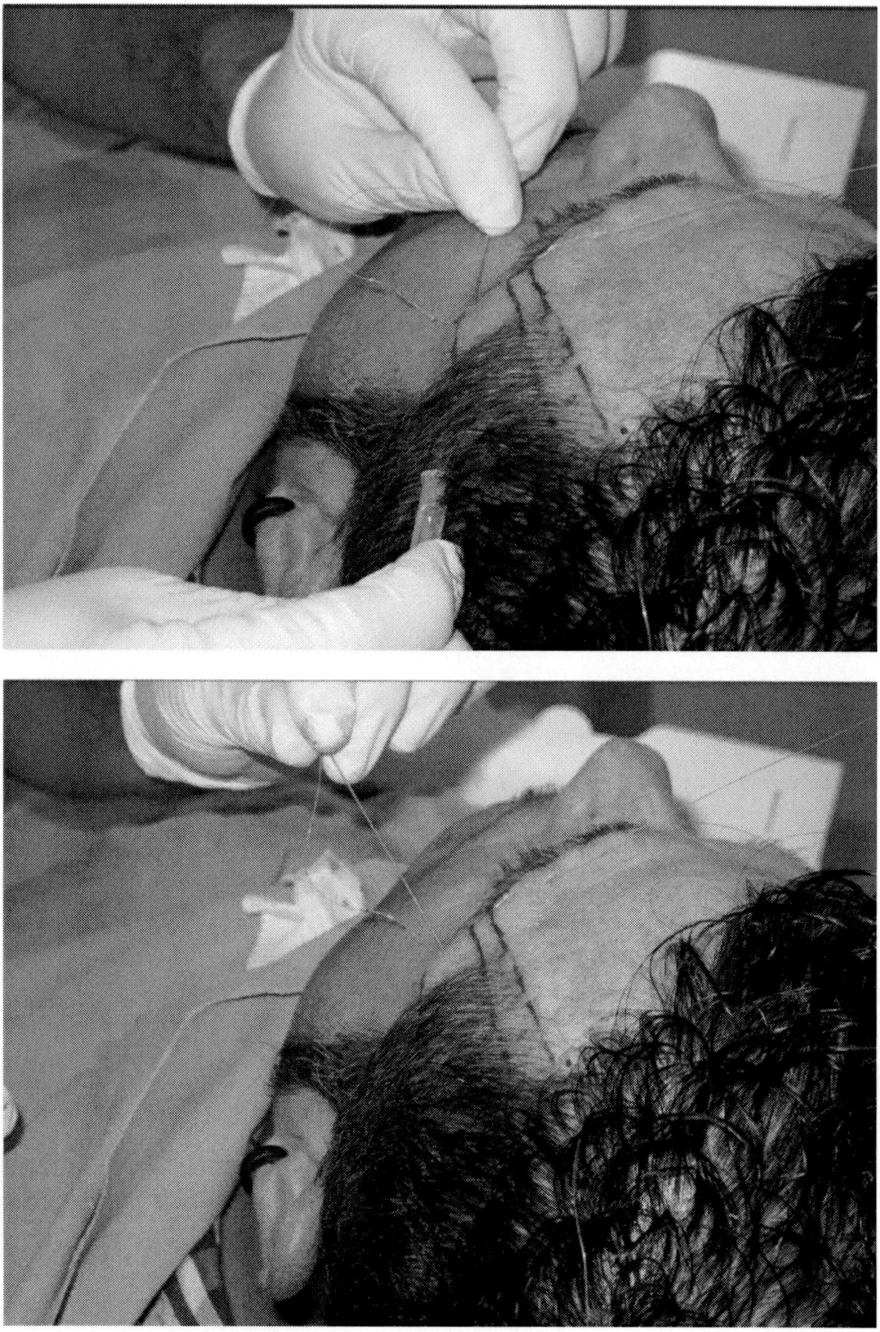

F. (Continued).

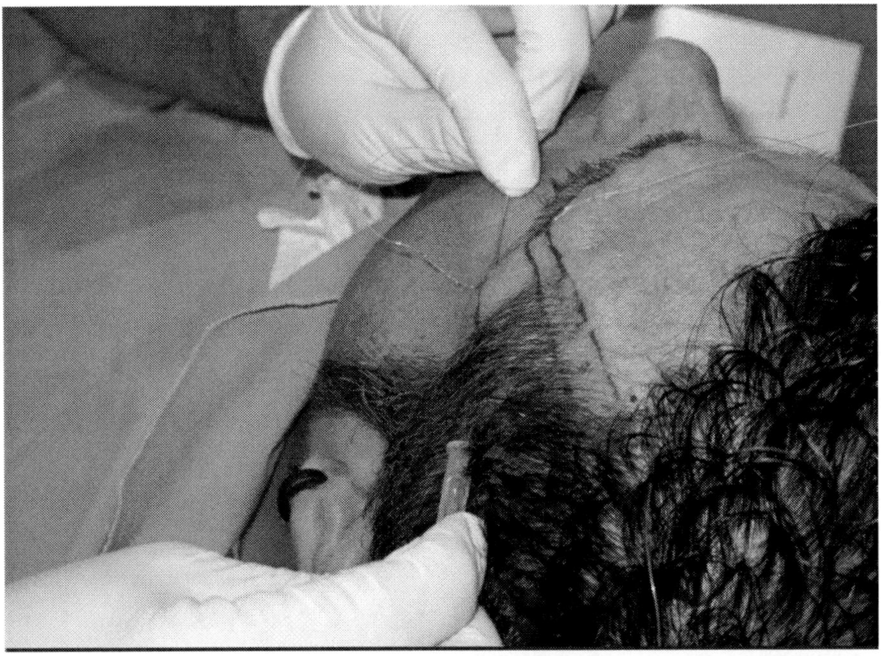

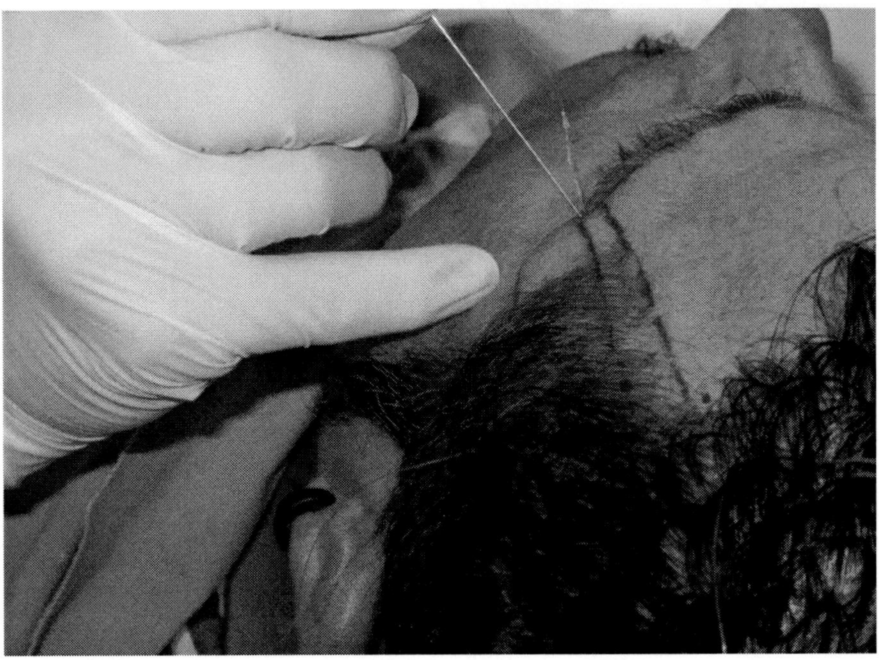

F. (Continued).

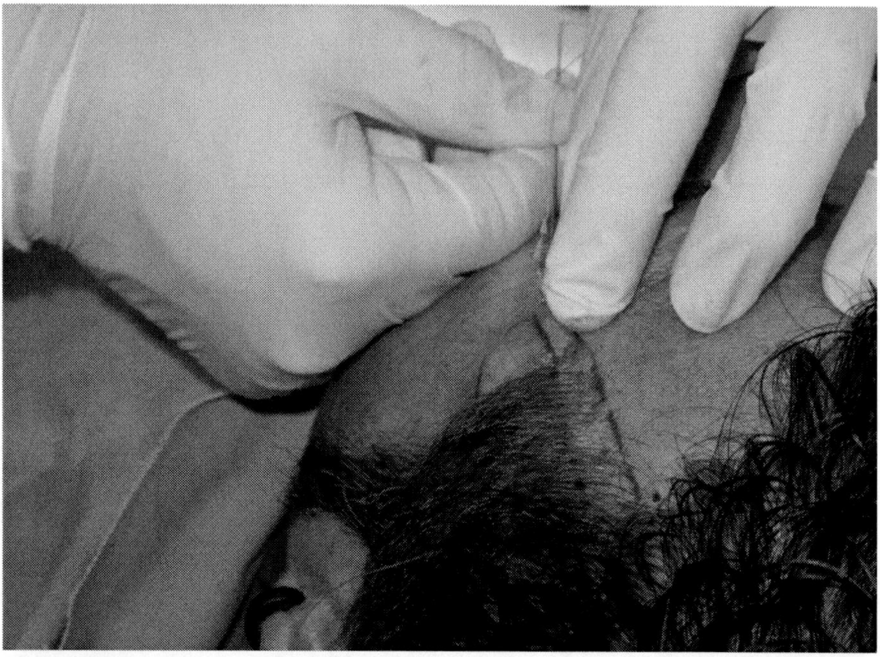

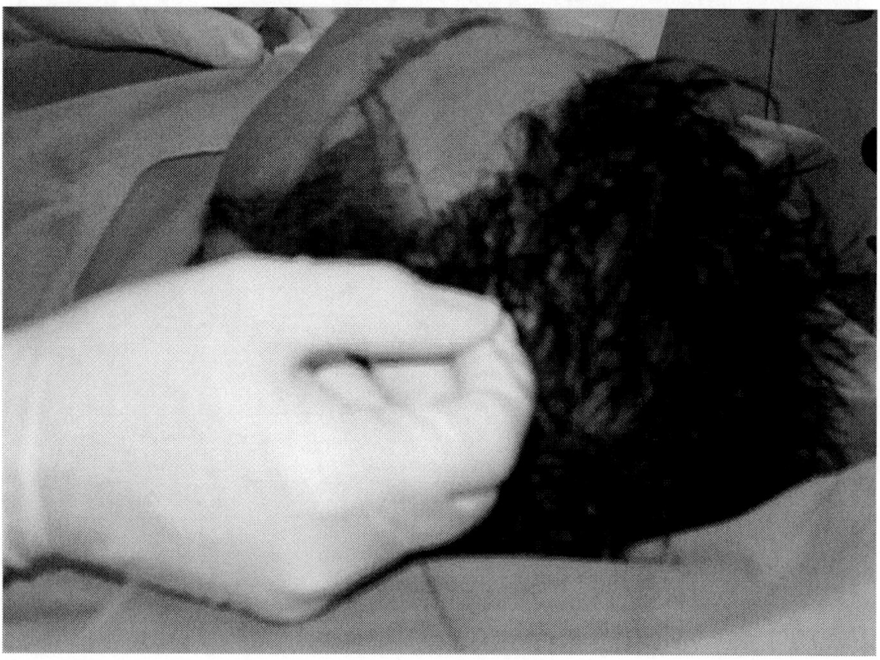

F. (Continued).

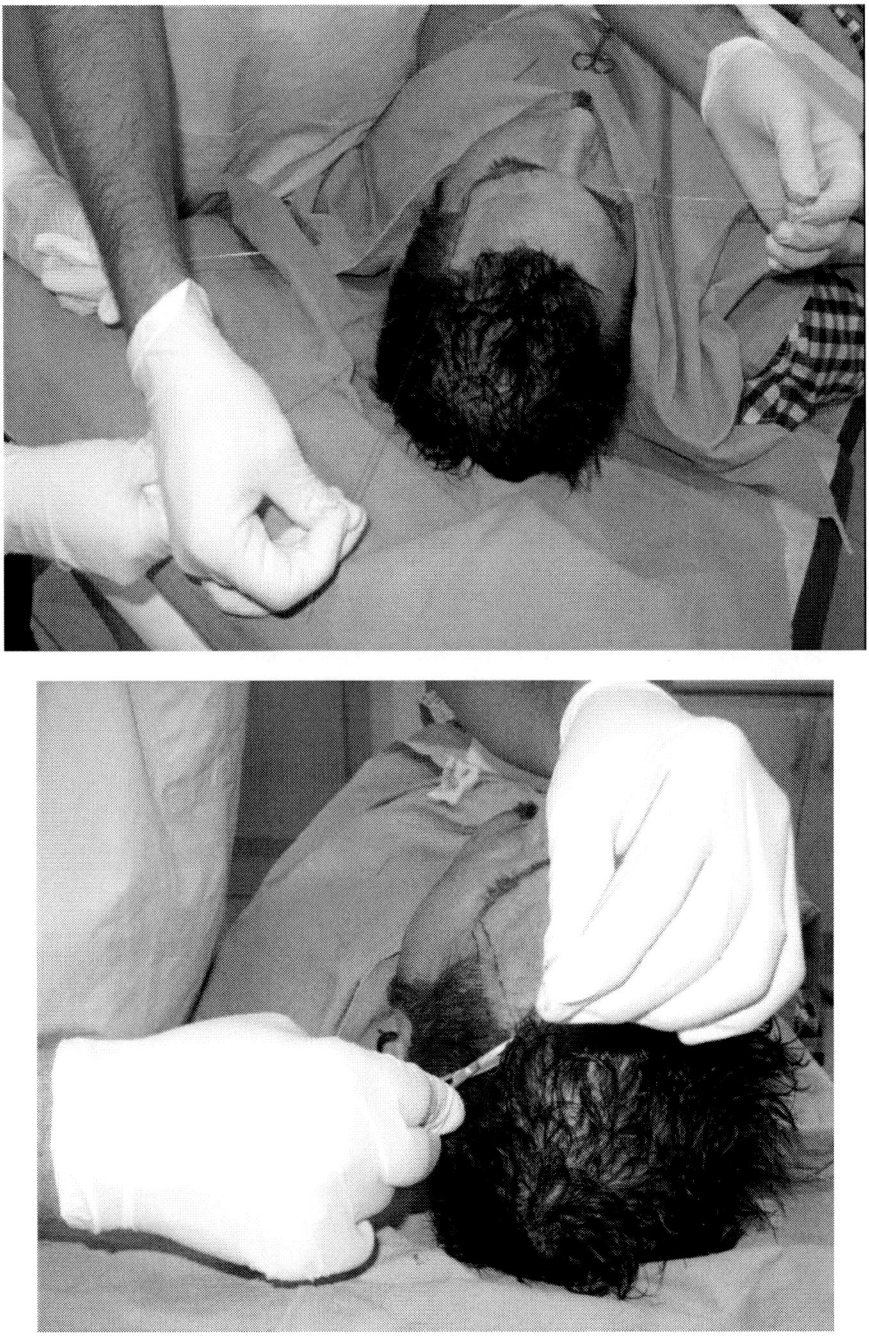

F. (Continued).

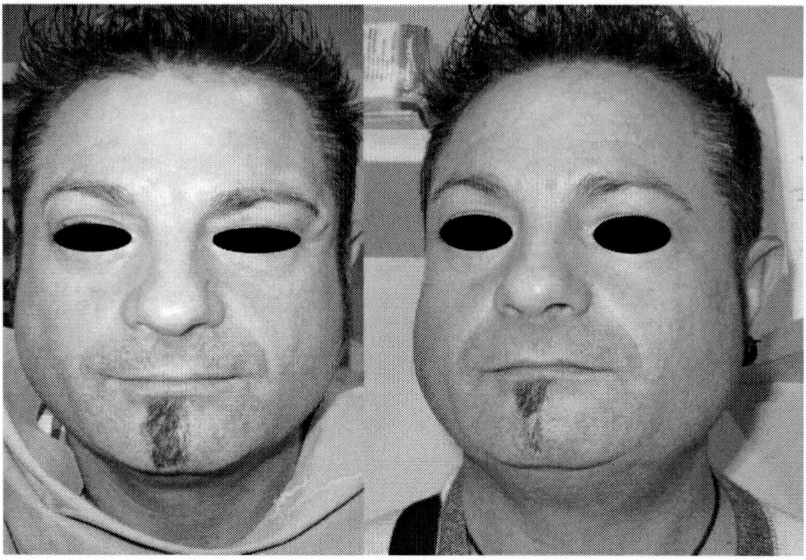

F: Multiple applications of coned wires to correct eyebrow asymmetry: project (1,2); injection of local anesthetic (3,4); the cutaneous plane is perforated by means of a 18 g needle (5); appropriate stripping of the wire (6) is needed before application; insertion of the guide needle for the first half of the first wire (7); the needle is the directed to the target point (8,9) and exits the cutaneous plane (10); insertion of the second half of the first wire (11-13); traction and tissue repositioning (14); for this very specific case we planned the central non coned part of the second wired to be hosted in a cutaneous tunnel to optimize traction: the tunnel is created by the usual 18 g needle (15-17), which is needed to allow precise insertion of the wire in the tunnel (18-21); guide needles are than used to insert the coned part of the wire in its two portions (22-24 and 25-27); traction and tissue repositioning (28); after the application the portion of the wires remaining out of the skin is removed by scissors (29); pre and postsurgical photos (30).

Results

All but two patients were satisfied with the outcomes after treatment. Subjective marks provided by patients ranked among “very good” (51 cases), “good” (73 cases), “fair” (5 cases), “bad” (2 cases). Consensus ratings by two independent surgeons found that objective outcomes were divided among “excellent”(in 53 cases), “good” (in 49 cases), and “fair” (in 29 cases). The postoperative course was uneventful except for trhree patients. Among these, 2 patients presented with major hematoma and another patient had minor skin dimpling. The two case with hematoma resolved spontaneously without any surgical interventions. The patient presenting the skin rippling needed surgical intervention to remove the wire.

Conclusion

The coned wire lift offers several advantages over classical approaches like surgical facial lifting.

Because of its semplicity it can be executed under simple local anesthesia. Surgical time is dramatically reduced, with great advantage for the surgeon and for the patient. The absence of skin incisions leads to immediate recovery and absence of visible scars.

This technique can be associated with filler or botulin toxin injections in the same surgical time, to optimize the aesthetic enhancement and reduce patient stress.

Index

A

D

E

Q

R

S

T